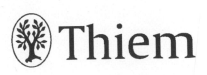

K-Wiring
Principles and Techniques

Second Edition

C. Rex, MS (Ortho), DNB (Ortho), FRCS (Ed.), FRCS (Tr & Ortho), MCh (Ortho) Liverpool, PhD, DSc (Ortho)
Chief Consultant Orthopedic and Trauma Surgeon
Head of Department of Orthopedics
Rex Ortho Hospital
Coimbatore, India

Thieme
Delhi • Stuttgart • New York • Rio de Janeiro

Publishing Director: Ritu Sharma
Development Editor: Dr Ambika Kapoor
Director-Editorial Services: Rachna Sinha
Project Manager: Gaurav Prabhuzantye
Vice President-Sales and Marketing: Arun Kumar Majji
Managing Director & CEO: Ajit Kohli

Thieme Medical and Scientific Publishers Private Limited
A 12, Second Floor, Sector 2, Noida 201 301,
Uttar Pradesh, India, +911204556600
Email: customerservice@thieme.in
www.thieme.in

Cover design: © Thieme
Cover image source: © Thieme

Page make-up by RECTO Graphics, India

Printed in India

5 4 3 2

ISBN 978-93-90553-62-4
Also available as an e-book:
eISBN 978-93-90553-63-1

Important note: Medicine is an ever-changing science undergoing continual development. Research and clinical experience are continually expanding our knowledge, in particular our knowledge of proper treatment and drug therapy. Insofar as this book mentions any dosage or application, readers may rest assured that the authors, editors, and publishers have made every effort to ensure that such references are in accordance with **the state of knowledge at the time of production of the book**.

Nevertheless, this does not involve, imply, or express any guarantee or responsibility on the part of the publishers in respect to any dosage instructions and forms of applications stated in the book. **Every user is requested to examine carefully** the manufacturers' leaflets accompanying each drug and to check, if necessary in consultation with a physician or specialist, whether the dosage schedules mentioned therein or the contraindications stated by the manufacturers differ from the statements made in the present book. Such examination is particularly important with drugs that are either rarely used or have been newly released on the market. Every dosage schedule or every form of application used is entirely at the user's own risk and responsibility. The authors and publishers request every user to report to the publishers any discrepancies or inaccuracies noticed. If errors in this work are found after publication, errata will be posted at www.thieme.com on the product description page.

Some of the product names, patents, and registered designs referred to in this book are in fact registered trademarks or proprietary names even though specific reference to this fact is not always made in the text. Therefore, the appearance of a name without designation as proprietary is not to be construed as a representation by the publisher that it is in the public domain.

Thieme addresses people of all gender identities equally. We encourage our authors to use gender-neutral or gender-equal expressions wherever the context allows.

This book, including all parts thereof, is legally protected by copyright. Any use, exploitation, or commercialization outside the narrow limits set by copyright legislation without the publisher's consent is illegal and liable to prosecution. This applies in particular to photostat reproduction, copying, mimeographing or duplication of any kind, translating, preparation of microfilms, and electronic data processing and storage.

Contents

Videos

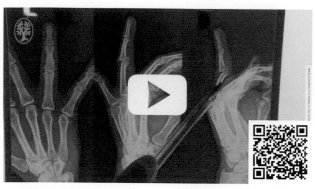

Video 2.1 Demonstration of dorsal blocking K-wire in volar plate avulsion fracture. https://www.thieme.de/de/q.htm?p=opn/cs/21/10/16821451-9a69b7c9

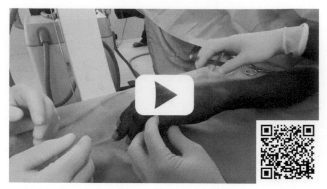

Video 2.3 Demonstration of base of the proximal phalanx fracture treated with antegrade K-wire. https://www.thieme.de/de/q.htm?p=opn/cs/21/10/16821415-ac2f1b53

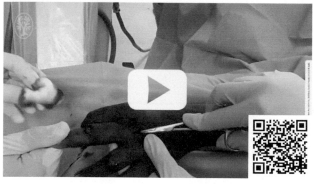

Video 2.2 Demonstration of reduction and fixation for neck of proximal phalanx fracture with K-wire. https://www.thieme.de/de/q.htm?p=opn/cs/21/10/16821414-543825b7

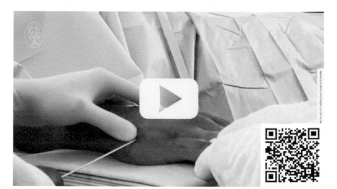

Video 2.4 Demonstration of metacarpal base fracture treated with two parallel K-wires. https://www.thieme.de/de/q.htm?p=opn/cs/21/10/16821416-94a117e4

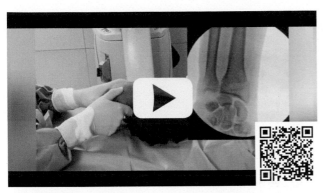

Video 3.1 Demonstration of distal-end radius fracture treated with three K-wires technique. https://www.thieme. de/de/q.htm?p=opn/cs/21/10/16821417-91b576a1

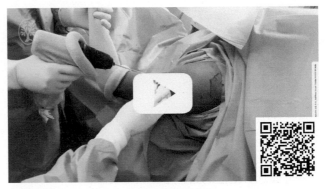

Video 7.1 Demonstration of four-part proximal humerus fracture reduced and fixed with K-wire. https://www.thieme. de/de/q.htm?p=opn/cs/21/10/16821419-2ce9bedf

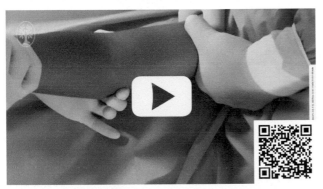

Video 5.1 Demonstration of supracondylar humerus fracture reduction and fixation with two cross K-wires. https:// www.thieme.de/de/q.htm?p=opn/cs/21/10/16821418-f97937e3

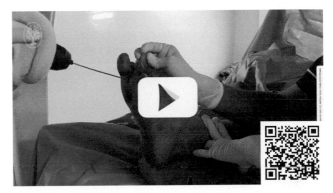

Video 14.1 Demonstration of K-wiring in multiple metatarsal fractures of foot. https://www.thieme.de/de/q. htm?p=opn/cs/21/10/16821420-85933e61

Foreword

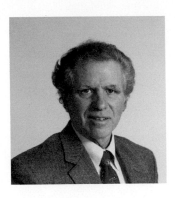

We continue to be seduced by technological "advances" in our fracture and reconstructive procedures, at times putting greater emphasis on the implant rather than its correct application. Yet the ubiquitous K-wire remains the workhorse of the surgeon regardless of the level of experience. Furthermore, the K-wire fulfills quite elegantly the requirements of a truly reliable implant. It is cost effective, can be used in virtually any health care center, does not require a "specialist" but rather any surgeon at any level of experience, and it is reliable with predictable results.

It comes as no surprise that the first edition of this book has been so successful, prompting the need for this second edition. Using more varied case examples, the reader will be impressed with the myriad applications of the K-wire. The pearls and pitfalls of its applications with step-by-step technical tips further expose one to the usefulness of this implant.

Any surgeon involved in the care of the hand and wrist will gain much from this text regardless of the level of experience. In fact, one will be exposed to more than a few applications and techniques which will be novel and further reveal the wonder of the K-wire.

With enthusiasm, I recommend that this text should be viewed by all members of one's department or institution.

Jesse B. Jupiter, MD
Past President, American Shoulder and Elbow Surgeons
Past President, American Association of Hand Surgeons
Emeritus Hansjoerg Wyss/AO Professor
Harvard Medical School
Visiting Orthopedic Surgeon
Massachusetts General Hospital
Boston, Massachusetts

Foreword

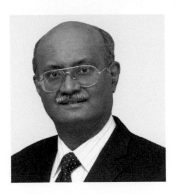

I am very happy to be invited to write the foreword for the second edition of the book by Dr. C. Rex on K-wires in orthopedics. When I wrote the foreword for the first edition, I had mentioned that K-wires were 'built to last,' as an implant for everyday use by any orthopedic surgeon. I had also mentioned that there was not a single book dealing with the history, science, and philosophy of the use of K-wires. Hence, it was predicted that this book, which fills that void, will be well received by surgeons and the student community. That prediction has been proven true when we see that this book has gone on to the second edition.

Dr. C. Rex has updated the text in various chapters and added new ones. These additions have been enumerated on the back cover of this book. They make this edition more valuable to the reader. As a hand surgeon, I use K-wires daily and they are used in surgical procedures as varied as from operating on a mallet finger to performing a hand replant. Though introducing K-wires may appear simple, successful outcome depends upon having a full understanding of the size of the wire to be used, the route of passing the wire, technical nuances to be followed, and knowledge on aftercare. That knowledge is important, and it will not be wrong if we say that as is our theory, so is our practice. This book is a great resource to provide all the information that is needed for good practice and achieving optimal outcomes.

I congratulate Dr. C. Rex in producing this second edition and wish its continued success.

S. Raja Sabapathy, MS, MCh, DNB (Plastic), FRCS (Ed.), FAMS, Hon FRCS (Glasgow), Hon FACS, DSc (Hon)
Chairman, Department of Plastic Surgery, Hand and Reconstructive Microsurgery and Burns
Director, Ganga Hospital
Coimbatore, India
President, Asian Pacific Federation of Societies for Surgery of the Hand (APFSSH)
Secretary General, International Federation of Societies for Surgery of the Hand (IFSSH)

Preface

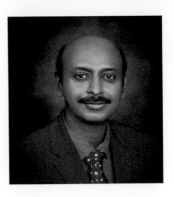

K-wire fixation is a subject of ignorance and little understanding without any clear conception of their role and performance. Executing K-wire fixation in small bones is very taxing or sometimes tougher than performing a tibial or femoral nailing. There is nothing like simple surgery in orthopedics, definitely not in terms of the size of the implant or the part of the body to be operated. A good planning will lead on to a well-executed surgery. For this, a thorough knowledge of the implant and its application is mandatory for good clinical practice.

There was an overwhelming response to the first edition of the book from all practicing orthopedic and hand surgeons, which necessitated the preparation of the second edition. This book is going to be a Holy book on the principles and techniques of K-wiring as it discusses the right indications, extended indications, avoidance of complications, and pitfalls, with respect to clinical application, with clear illustrative examples. Although K-wiring has evolved as a foremost implant more than a century ago, its application in clinical practice has changed considerably. It was designed initially for external traction, which was subsequently aimed for fixation of small, long bones of hand and foot.

Modern orthopedics includes the use of a plethora of newer implants and instrumentation but the K-wire has definitely stood the test of time and has many indications today in orthopedic and trauma practice. We have standardized the ways of K-wiring to be practiced for the best clinical outcome. Perfect placement of K-wire in phalanges can be challenging and suboptimal fixation can be avoided by mastering the surgical technique with proprioception and the feel, in addition to image intensifier guidance. In this book, the safe corridor for the entry of K-wire in the hand is described, and the associated tips and tricks are discussed. In this second edition, more clear concepts on this type of fixation have been added with additional case scenarios demonstrating the utilization of different ways of fixation. It covers A to Z on the usage of K-wire from fingertip to toes. We have described K-wire utilization in an exhaustive manner including the postoperative regime. I am sure this book will be an enriching manual for practical guidance and quick reference in an orthopedic trauma theater. Not only is it a cost-cutting surgical procedure, minimally invasive, freely available in any part of the world, both rural and urban, has less inventory, etc., but it is also surgeon friendly in many situations when other options have failed. I am thankful to all my teachers, my colleagues, and the readers for making this a successful endeavor, and a reference book destined to last as long as the implant "K-wire" exists.

C. Rex, MS (Ortho), DNB (Ortho), FRCS (Ed.), FRCS (Tr & Ortho), MCh (Ortho) Liverpool, PhD, DSc (Ortho)

Acknowledgments

I am extremely thankful to the Rex Ortho Hospital management, theater staff, and departmental workers whose cooperation and encouragement have made this possible. My special thanks to my student, Dr. Shylendra Babu, who is presently a junior consultant in our team, for compiling and correcting the manuscript with his smiling face and dedicated effort throughout. His contribution is commendable.

I am thankful to our specialty consultants, Dr. Premanand, Dr. Harish Kumar, and Dr. Sathish Kumar, and all our alumni who have directly or indirectly helped me in preparing this book. I am grateful to my anesthesia colleagues, Dr. Palaniappan, Dr. Venkatesh, Dr. Prasanth, and Dr. Jaikrishnan, who have helped me in taking photographs during the surgical procedures. I thank Dr. Amith Ram and Ram Prasad for their helping hand in preparation. I am thankful to my patients without whom this venture would not have been possible. I am thankful to my father, Dr. M. Chandrabose, Managing Director of Rex Ortho Hospital, for his continuous encouragement. Last but not the least, I thank my mother, my family, and all my well-wishers who have influenced me in writing this book and making this mission complete.

C. Rex, MS (Ortho), DNB (Ortho), FRCS (Ed.), FRCS (Tr & Ortho), MCh (Ortho) Liverpool, PhD, DSc (Ortho)

1 K-Wire

History

In 1909, Martin Kirschner (1879–1942) introduced a smooth pin, now known as the Kirschner wire (K-wire). The K-wire was initially used for skeletal traction but is now used for many different goals. The development of the K-wire and its insertion devices were mainly influenced by the change in operative goals and the introduction of antibiotics. Despite these reasons, the K-wire is now standard for the treatment of hand fractures worldwide.

Martin Kirschner was born on 28th October 1879 in Breslau, Germany, now known as Wroclaw, Poland. He studied medicine in Freiburg, Zurich, and Munich, and received his MD degree from the University of Strasbourg, France in 1904. In 1909 Kirschner introduced one of his most important contributions to emergency medicine, that is, thick, smooth pins that evolved over the years into thin, smooth, stainless steel (SS) wires with various tips. The latter are now known as K-wires. It took quite some years for the K-wire to evolve into its current feature. The development was influenced by various factors, such as wound infection, refinement of the insertion method, and change of its goals; for example, it became more useful for the small fragile bones than the thick long bones. During his lifetime, Kirschner was promoted to professor of surgery at the University of Konigsberg (East Prussia), the University of Tubingen (Germany), and the University of Heidelberg (Germany) in 1916, 1927, and 1934, respectively. He remained at Heidelberg until his death, on 30th August 1942, due to an inoperable carcinoma of the stomach.

Initially, the K-wire was a pin and not a wire, which Kirschner used for "Nagel extension (nail extension)," that is, skeletal traction for fractures of the long bones by means of a nail. The principle of the pin was based on the Steinmann nail, which was introduced by Fritz Steinmann in 1907. Steinmann placed two nails in the distal fragment of a broken bone, laterally and medially; thereafter traction was applied to the protruding ends of the nails, thus keeping the fragments in proper alignment. In contrast to Steinmann, Kirschner placed only one pin throughout the distal end of the fractured bone; it was hammered through a predrilled hole. The pins Kirschner used had a diamond-shaped tip and diameters varying from 3.5 to 6.0 mm—today, they are surprisingly known as Steinmann pins. Throughout the years it became more and more obvious that the Steinmann pins often resulted in infection. According to both Steinmann and Kirschner, these infections were due to thickness of the pins and thus the necessity of predrilling, which resulted in to-and-fro slipping of the pin. Therefore, Kirschner refined and improved an insertion apparatus that made it possible to insert small-diameter wires without predrilling, which resulted in a diminished rate of infection. In 1927, he showed his external accordion-like guide that made it possible to insert thin chromium-plated steel piano wires, varying in diameter from 0.7 to 1.5 mm, without the need of predrilling. From that moment on, K-wires could be driven percutaneously through the skin, soft tissue, and bone. As predrilling was no longer necessary, the wire was rigidly seated within the bone, so that lateral slipping was avoided, as well as trauma to the soft tissues. Kirschner called the procedure "Draht extension (wire extension)" instead of "Nagel extension." The external accordion-like wire guide could be combined with a hand drill or a power drill. It was, however, difficult to handle. This resulted in the development of an improved and simpler K-wire drill by Mathews in 1931. Nowadays we have cannulated K-wire motorized drivers with quick release for easy insertion and handling.

From 1935 other indications for the K-wire were described, such as maintaining reduction of fracture-dislocations of the ankle joint, the hip, and the elbow. In 1937, the use of K-wires was advocated for the treatment of hand fractures, which is the main purpose they are used for today.

In World War II, surgeons became progressively more innovative in the use of K-wires because of the introduction of antibiotics and corrosion-resistant metals. K-wires with a diameter of 1.5 mm were generally used in World War II, and thinner ones (0.7–1.0 mm) were used for the fingers. In 1940, Murray started to place K-wires in a relatively new manner, longitudinally through the medullary cavity of the clavicle. His enthusiasm pushed him to extend this intramedullary technique to the radius, the ulna, and the fibula. This new technique was applied to metacarpal fractures; this treatment was very useful in the army where patients could be assigned to light duty immediately after surgery. Today the K-wire is universally used in hand fractures and for many other indications such as foot and ankle surgery, long-bone fractures in children and adults, pelvic fractures, treatment of Buerger disease, phalloplasty during female-to-male transsexual surgery, and stabilization of costal cartilage in nasal surgery to prevent wrapping.[1]

Besides the changes in K-wire insertion devices, the K-wire itself has changed over the years. In 1909, the original K-wire had a diamond-shaped tip. Over the past three decades, research has been done regarding K-wire characteristics such as tip and diameter (**Fig. 1.1**). The most frequently analyzed K-wire tips are the diamond (flat) and trocar (pyramid-shaped). The trocar tip needs the highest insertion force, resulting in a significantly higher temperature development compared with the diamond tip, but it results in a significantly better fixation, especially immediately after insertion. In 1999 a newly designed tip was proposed: it had two steep flutes for the removal of bone fragments during drilling; this tip provoked the lowest temperature elevations during insertion, as compared with the trocar and diamond tip.

Another important K-wire characteristic is the diameter. K-wires with diameters smaller than 1.1 mm generate more heat than thicker K-wires, regardless of the tip configuration. In addition to smooth K-wires regularly used in hand surgery, there are fine-threaded K-wires used for shoulder, foot, and ankle surgery. These threaded K-wires need significantly more extraction force than smooth K-wires, and they must be removed by anticlockwise rotation movement rather than pulling. Threaded K-wires can prevent migration and have better purchase in osteoporotic bone.

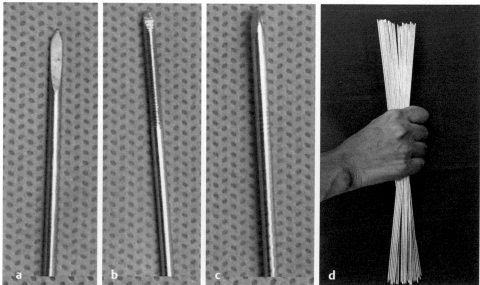

Fig. 1.1 (a–d) Different K-wire tips.

[1] Franssen BB, Schuurman AH, Van der Molen AM, Kon M. One century of Kirschner wires and Kirschner wire insertion techniques: a historical review. Acta Orthop Belg 2010;76(1):1–6.

In his final article, Kirschner discussed the disadvantages of drilling K-wires, such as wire migration and pin tract infection, and he wondered how to prevent these and finally mentioned the insertion of K-wires by hammering instead of drilling. He even described and produced a hammer device that he called the "Drahtnagler." He stressed that hammering prevented heat development, which resulted in a longer and better fixation. K-wires with a diameter of 1.5 mm were used for this hammer device.

To minimize the high heat produced by power drills, some hand surgeons recommend drilling K-wires by the hand whenever possible, but it compromises on the precision work. The surgical wires (316LVM SS, 304V SS, nitinol [nickel titanium, NiTi]) used to manufacture K-wires are of medical-grade quality for temporary fixation during the surgery or for temporary surgical implantation that only remains throughout the required time of healing. Material selection is often based on personal preferences. However, because of the cost differences between SS and NiTi and their clinical applications, SS is favored. SS wires develop a highly polished appearance when drawn to fine diameters. The surface of smaller diameters (sized 0.040 in or less) can be further smoothened using single crystal natural diamond dies.

Material Properties

Stainless Steel 316LVM Wire

SS 316LVM is a medical-grade steel that is vacuum-melted for purity. It is used for implantable medical devices, and is also applicable for fabricating components for precision electronics and the fabrication of woven wire cloth. This small-diameter wire has a chemical composition that consists of Cr, Ni, Mo, and Mn. The 316LVM SS wire is a suitable close-tolerance material used in fabricating custom K-wires to our exact tolerance specifications.

Stainless Steel 304V Wire

This medical-grade, austenitic SS wire is initially electric-arc–melted. For purity and homogeneity, the metal is further refined with vacuum-arc melting. The typical chemical composition of SS 304V may include Cr, Ni, C, Mn, Mo, Si, P, Cu, Co, and N. Being one of the least expensive medical materials, it is the most popular alloy for medical appliances. Not only does it have an excellent strength, but it is also easy to weld. Besides K-wires, other common medical device components using the SS 304V alloy include guide wires, stylets, needles, and catheters.

Nitinol Wire

Medical grade titanium is generally accepted as an optimal material for implantable devices because of its extreme tolerance by surrounding contact tissues, and it does not induce toxic or inflammatory reactions. The good biocompatibility is thought to be due to the stable titanium oxide layer.

Clinical Application in Fracture Fixation

Fracture fixation with K-wire can be of two types.

Direct Fracture Fixation

- Transosseous interfragmentary short purchase fixation: This is practiced in periarticular or metaphyseal fracture fixation. For example, distal radius fracture fixation, supracondylar fracture fixation, unicondylar fracture of phalanges, patella, and olecranon fracture fixation with supplementary tension band stainless steel wire.
- Transosseous intramedullary long purchase fixation: This is practiced in shaft fractures of short long bones or long bones of extremities. For example, metacarpal or metatarsal shaft fracture fixation, proximal phalanx fracture, pediatric both bones forearm fractures, and humerus shaft in a child.

Indirect Fracture Fixation

Most of the partial intra-articular fracture with joint dislocation or subluxation the primary importance is given to joint reduction and congruity. A joint transfixation K-wire will suffice to treat and maintain the fracture fragments. For example, Bennett's fracture dislocation, volar plate avulsion fracture with dorsal blocking K-wire, and mallet finger.

K-wire used to buttress the fracture as in intrafocal pinning in distal radius fracture (Kapandji technique) and bony mallet finger fixation is another example.

Pros and Cons of K-Wire Fixation

One of the advantages of the K-wire is the relative ease of insertion with minimal trauma to the soft tissue and the tendons; however, its greatest advantage is the possibility of atraumatic percutaneous insertion. This technique is easier than open reduction and internal fixation, has less associated risks, minimizes swelling and stiffness, and is still preferred today. Percutaneous K-wire fixation achieves stable fixation after adequate reduction and allows early mobilization in order to prevent permanent deformity and stiffness.

Percutaneous K-wire fixation diminishes and even avoids complications that occur after open reduction and internal fixation, including infection, difficulties in fracture healing, stiffness due to extensive soft tissue dissection, fibrosis, extensor tendon adhesion, plate loosening or breakage, and complex regional pain syndrome. Intramedullary K-wire fixation is even simpler and puts the least strain on the muscles and tendons.

However, K-wires have their drawbacks too. The first article that appeared in 1939 discouraged the use of K-wires, describing their migration and lack of rigidity and strength when used in femoral neck fractures. In 1943, the first cases of K-wire migration from the clavicle to the lungs were reported. K-wire migration still occurs today and is a serious problem because it can result in nonfatal to devastating complications and even death. In most of the reported cases the K-wires migrated from the shoulder girdle to the aorta, heart, lung, trachea, mediastinum, neck, spleen, and spinal canal. There are also reports of migration from other anatomical sites such as from the hip to the heart, liver, or popliteal fossa, and even from the left hand into the heart. The explanation of the K-wire migration remains obscure, but in most cases migration can be prevented by bending the distal end of the K-wire. Nevertheless, even bent wires can migrate after breakage, so follow-up radiographs should be made until the K-wires are removed.

Pin tract infections have occurred ever since the introduction of the K-wire. This complication was one of the factors which resulted in the development of thinner K-wires. However, even with smaller-diameter K-wires, pin tract infections still occur. Drilling too many times to get the desired position is one of the reasons for infection and this complication becomes less with surgeon's experience.

A system of sterile dressing covered with foam rubber padding was placed where the K-wire penetrates the skin. This can be used to prevent skin necrosis and infection. The incidence of pin tract infections should not be underestimated. At present, the use of K-wire results in pin tract infections in 2.2 to 21% of the cases. This complication may lead to earlier pin removal and thus to nonunion. Early treatment of pin tract infection is important, either by immobilization, antibiotics, or removal of loose pins. Fewer infections are seen when K-wires are buried, but it necessitates another procedure of removal in theater rather than an outpatient procedure and thus chance of migration is greater.

Other complications described through the years are damage to peripheral structures such as rupture of the tendons, traumatic subarachnoid-pleural fistula, and toxic shock. Restriction of active motion until the wires are removed can result in diminished function after bone healing.

Therefore, the most important goal is to further minimize these complications by adequate cooling during drilling, bending the protruding ends, or if possible burying the wires as and when necessary, such as in patients with diabetes or in a fracture fixation that may take long time to heal.

Indications for K-Wire in Orthopedics

K-wire is a straight SS wire of varying thickness from 0.75 to 4.0 mm in diameter. It is neither too flexible as SS wire nor too rigid as an intramedullary nail. It has various applications in orthopedics as follows:

- K-wire is used in fixation of small-bone fractures and fracture dislocations in the hand and feet by transfixing with bicortical purchase or single intramedullary wire placement across the fracture or stacking with multiple intramedullary K-wires for stability and strength in short long-bone fixations (e.g., metacarpal, metatarsal, and clavicle) and sometimes behaving like a flexible nail in pediatric long-bone intramedullary fixations.

- It is used for transfixing and maintaining the reduction of unstable joint dislocations and open dislocations.
- It is used for fusion of small joints (e.g., arthrodesis of interphalangeal joints).
- It is used as a splint for soft tissue healing and plastic procedures (e.g., mallet finger, open-finger injuries, heel flap avulsion).
- It is used for maintenance in deformity correction (e.g., club foot corrective surgeries) and contracture corrections.
- It is used as a temporary fixation during fracture reduction in periarticular fractures, in butterfly fragment fixation, and in comminuted fractures to aid reduction before stabilizing with a definitive implant.
- It is used in fixation of malunion and nonunion fractures of small bones.
- It is used for stabilizing excision arthroplasty (e.g., claw toe, hammer toe deformity correction, Keller arthroplasty, trapeziectomy, etc.).
- K-wire can be used as drill to pass suture anchors in shoulder surgery, pass nylon wires through the tract for pullout stitches on drilling distal phalanx, and to pass straight needle with nylon (e.g., mallet finger).
- It is an immense tool for drilling exposed subchondral bone in arthroscopy in knee and ankle for microfracture. As the wire is flexible, it does not easily break on drilling unlike the drill bits.
- It can also serve as a drill for insertion of locking bolts in intramedullary nailing. In distal humerus anteroposterior interlocking screw placement, K-wire gives much safety in drilling without tethering major neurovascular structures unlike a drill bit. It also helps in distal femur/tibia interlocking screw entry point where one has made several entries with drill bit and where it is difficult to change the entry point in a slopping surface or on a bony ridge or because of preexisting hole. It is a useful technique for beginners to centralize in the interlocking screw hole and mark with a K-wire entry before using a proper drill for locking screw placement to prevent slippage.
- K-wire is used as a guiding tool for passing another implant, such as in cannulated screw fixations, and for positioning of implants such as locking plates (**Figs. 1.2** and **1.3**).

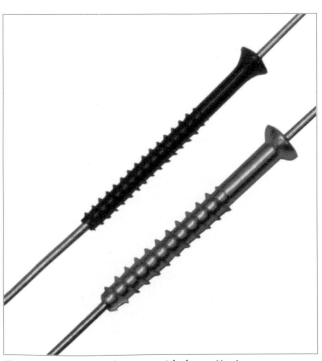

Fig. 1.2   Cannulated screw guided on a K-wire.

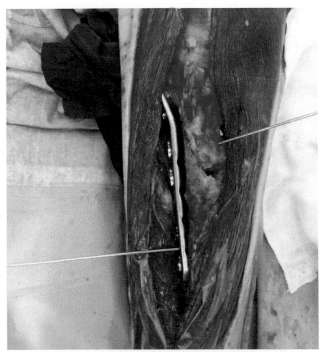

Fig. 1.3   A K-wire used to stabilize the long oblique fracture and another K-wire used to position the locking plate.

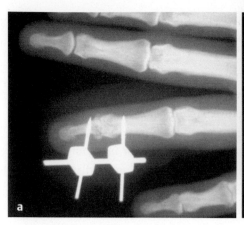
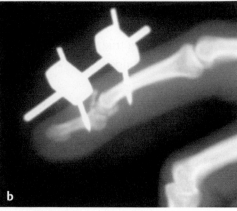

Fig. 1.4 (a, b) K-wire used to transfix the bone and attached to a special clamp on unilateral external fixator rod.

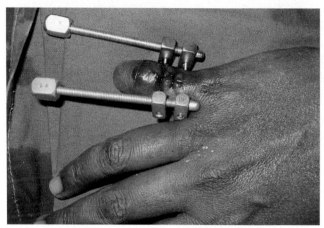

Fig. 1.5 K-wire transfixing the bone attached to dual-frame external fixator for distraction osteogenesis.

- It is used as an appliance in K-wire traction, in Ilizarov fixation, and as a transfixing pin in external fixator for phalanx fractures as shown in **Figs. 1.4 to 1.7**.
- It can also be used as an identification marker or as a reference in C-arm scan for proper placement of implant (e.g., placement of dynamic condylar screw or angled blade plate in the distal femur, in spine pedicle, and level identification).
- K-wire is used to retract soft tissues especially in lateral exposure of calacaneum. The thick lateral calcaneal flap is retracted away from the working spot by inserting two K-wires into talus to keep soft tissue flap retracted up. It is also used in retracting abductor muscles in exposure of the acetabulum by lateral approach.

- For appropriate positioning of a plate (especially LCP): K-wires can be used for positioning the plate, through the hole provided in the plate for the same or just anterior or posterior to the plate to act as a stopper beyond which the plate cannot slide or more before definitive screw placement.
- K-wire can be used to remove the overgrown bone in the plate (especially over the corners and margins of a plate) and screw heads as a drill before implant removal. Also using a K-wire to drill the bone around the partially threaded screw is safer than a drill bit in view of drill bit breakage for removal of the implant.
- K-wire is used to break the bonding in uncemented femoral component removal by drilling multiple K-wires all around the stem between the prosthesis bone interface to break the bone ingrowth and ongrowth in revision hip surgeries.
- Apart from operating table usage, K-wire is also used as an instrument to clean the cannulated drills, drill bits, cannulated screw drivers, disc punches, rongeurs, and curettes. It is also used to remove blockage of the cannulated instruments, suction tubes, and vents. K-wire is a useful tool for removing the bone debris/impacted guide wire from a cannulated drill bit.
- K-wire in combination with special K-wire retractor device can be used to distract and provide adequate work space during foot fusion surgeries and to prepare for cage placement in cervical spine surgeries.

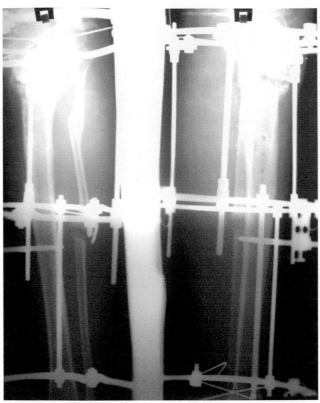

Fig. 1.6 Long cross K-wires through the bone attached to Ilizarov ring fixator after tensioning.

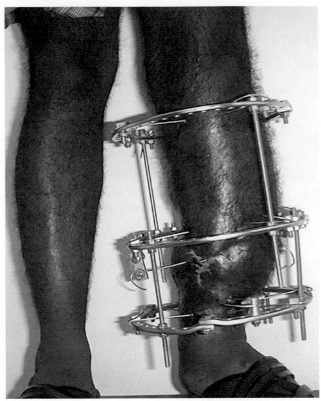

Fig. 1.7 Ilizarov ring fixator with tensioned K-wires used in the infected nonunion tibia.

K-Wire Used in External Fixator

K-wires are used to transfix the bone segments and to attach to the external fixator. It is used in hand fractures as shown in **Fig. 1.4** either as a unilateral frame fixation or double-frame external fixator (**Fig. 1.5**). Thin K-wires of 0.8, 1, or 1.2 mm are used in hand surgery for this purpose.

Long thin tip K-wires of 1.8 mm diameter are used in tension to transfix the long bones in ring fixators such as Ilizarov frame in divergent configuration as shown in **Figs. 1.6** and **1.7**.

K-Wire for Retracting Soft Tissues

Minimally invasive percutaneous plate osteosynthesis (MIPPO) for a tibial plateau facture through small anterolateral incision was done to slide the plate. The K-wire was drilled on the posterior cortex of tibia for retracting the tibialis anterior muscle and the skin flap posteriorly

for better visualization (**Fig. 1.8**) and the plate along the submuscular plane in correct position (**Fig. 1.9**).

Similarly K-wire is used to retract the calcaneal flap by passing the wire on talus to keep it away from the calcaneum for better exposure in lateral approach for internal fixation of calcaneum (**Fig. 1.9**).

K-Wire Retractor

K-wires as a component of special spreaders/retractors are used in the small bones, such as in foot surgery, to distract the joint after the insertion of K-wire (2.5 or 1.5 mm) in the individual bones to visualize the joint and to prepare for fusion. Small laminar spreaders destroy the edges especially in osteoporotic bones, which can be avoided by this special instrument. This technique is also used in cervical spine body distraction for preparation of intervertebral disk space and insertion of titanium cage for fixation (**Figs. 1.10a, b** and **1.11a–d**).

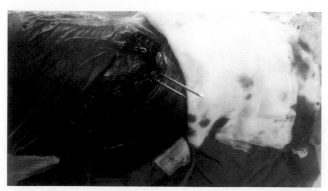

Fig. 1.8 Two K-wires inserted along the posterolateral border of tibia to retract the anterolateral muscles.

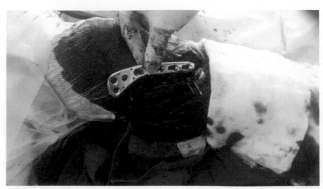

Fig. 1.9 Plate osteosynthesis (MIPPO) for a tibial plateau fracture through small anterolateral incision was done to slide the plate.

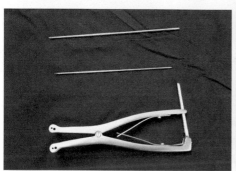
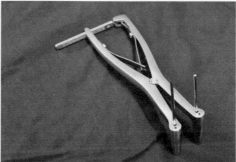

Fig. 1.10 **(a, b)** K-wire distractor instrument using K-wire to distract the joint

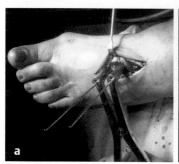
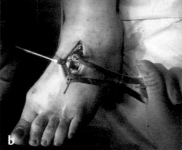
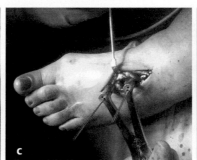
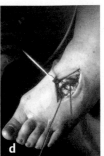

Fig. 1.11 **(a–d)** K-wire used as a spreader with the special distraction instrument in midtarsal fusion.

Inventory

K-wires of various lengths and diameters are available with either smooth or threaded ends as listed here:

- Tip:
  - ➢ Trocar end.
  - ➢ Diamond end.
- Diameter:
  - ➢ 0.75 to 5 mm.
- Length:
  - ➢ 15 to 30 cm.

Fig. 1.12 shows a quick coupling pneumatic K-wire driver, multipurpose nose plier, wire cutter, and wire bender, which are the basic instruments necessary for the performance of the surgical procedure. The AO K-wire (AO Foundation, Davos, Switzerland) drill sleeve has been shown separately, which can be used in placing adjacent parallel K-wires (**Fig. 1.13a, b**). Different sizes of K-wires applied in different types of bones are depicted in **Table 1.1**.

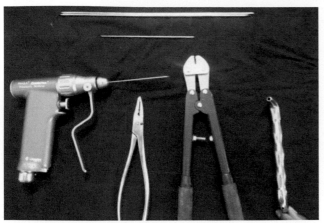

Fig. 1.12 Instruments used in application of K-wire: a cannulated drill, nose plier, wire cutter, and wire bender.

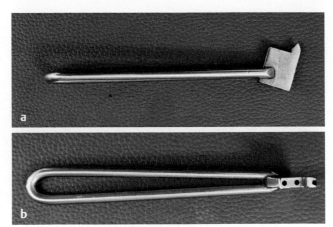

Fig. 1.13 (a, b) K-wire drill sleeve.

Table 1.1 Size of K-wires used in different types of bones

Site	K-wire size
Clavicle	2.5/3 mm
Acromioclavicular joint	2/2.5 mm
Proximal humerus	2.5/2.7 mm threaded tip or guide wire
Supracondylar humerus	1.5/2/2.2 mm depending on the age and bone size
Distal radius	2/2.5 mm
Scaphoid	1.5/1.8 mm
Metacarpal/Metatarsal	1.8/2 mm
Proximal phalanx (hand and feet)	1.5/1.8 mm
Middle phalanx	1.2/1.5 mm
Distal phalanx	1/1.2 mm
Ankle medial malleolus fracture	1.8/2 mm
Ankle lateral malleolus intramedullary	Isthmus diameter in distal fibula 1.5 to 3 mm
Ankle tibiocalcaneal pin	4 mm/5 mm

General Technique

An appropriate-sized K-wire for a particular bone or a purpose is selected as described in **Table 1.1** and also described in each section. The working length of the wire on the drill bit attachment should not be too long (from tip of the K-wire to drill attachment); as the wire is flexible, it may wobble or bend during drilling. For a precise work, the working length should be short, which makes the K-wire implant rigid to drill on the bone. Quick coupling K-wire drivers are very helpful for this purpose.

For a retrograde wiring technique, K-wires with sharpness on both ends should be used for drilling.

Generally, on piercing the far cortex with K-wire, one should immediately stop to make it not too proud, in order to prevent impalement of soft tissues. Pulling back after piercing the bone loosens the fixation with poor pullout strength. The feel of piercing the bone and checking with C-arm with gentle progression are important to stop the wire at the desired final position without reversing back.

Another important rule while bending the K-wire is to ensure that no force is transmitted to K-wire by holding with a wire holder or plier. The nose plier is kept flush to the bone/soft tissue and a 90-degree bent is given. It may suddenly rotate or twist or pull out while bending the wire. The wire is bent perpendicular to the holding plier and not sideways as it may rotate. It is bent 3 mm away from the nose plier with the wire bender or metal suction nozzle as bending very close to the nose plier will sometimes pull out the wire by few millimeters (the bender acts like a long lever arm and fulcrum at the bending point, abuts against the plier, and levers it out). Once the wire is bent, it is desirable not to twist or turn the K-wire as this may again make it loose. Therefore, the final position of bent wire should be analyzed and bent in that direction. Further, 90-degree bent is done to make it like a hook.

Thermal necrosis of bone from drilling with thick wire can be minimized by saline irrigation on open K-wiring procedures, and in closed percutaneous procedures. Betadine (Purdue Products L.P., Stamford, CT) painting on the wire helps in lubrication, reducing thermal necrosis and infection.

At the end of the procedure the pin wound is irrigated with normal saline to remove any bone debris and dressed with Jelonet and a Betadine-soaked foam pad in order to prevent infection.

On applying multiple adjacent K-wires, it is a good habit to protect the tip of the K-wire, outside in the space from pricking the surgeon's or assistant's hand or eyes, by covering with a needle sheath or a rubber wrap as shown in **Fig. 1.14**.

Bending the K-wire more than 90 degrees and leaving 1 to 2 cm long from the bend is essential in order to prevent migration or getting buried under the skin. If one wants to bend the wire to almost 170 to 180 degrees, as in case of wire buried under the skin or transfixation

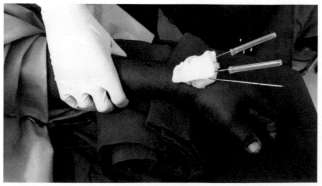

Fig. 1.14 A needle sheath or a rubber wrap can be used to protect the tip of the K-wire injuring the surgeon.

K-wire abutting the bone surface, the following technic can be used.

K-Wire Bending Technique

Buried K-wires under the skin are bent as close as 170 to 180 degrees to prevent soft tissue impalement and also to punch the K-wire close to the bone after a good bend at the end. This is important in K-wire used for fixing medial malleolus, lateral malleolus, patella, olecranon, etc. If one wants more acute hair-pin bend of K-wire, the following technique is useful. Here the first bend was given by holding with nose plier and a K-wire bender was used to get just more than 90-degree angle. A second bend was given by holding with pointed nose plier just distal to the first bend, and exactly in opposite direction, bending was done to just more than 90 degrees. This gives a "Z"-like appearance. Now holding the K-wire with nose plier close to the pin bone surface, the K-wire bender was used to bend in the opposite direction which makes the first bend to increase the angle to almost 160 to 180 degrees. The only disadvantage of this technique is that the K-wire can rotate during the maneuver of bending, making it loose. It is not advisable in osteoporotic bone or if the wire is too thick (**Fig. 1.15a–g**).

In tension band wiring, once the K-wire crosses the far cortex, pull it back by 5 mm from its final position using the K-wire driver. This prevents overpenetration through the second cortex (on the opposite side of the bone) after the wire is bent and impacted into place.

Complications from K-Wiring

No procedure is without complications. The common problems encountered due to K-wiring are as follows.

Loss of Fixation

Loss of fixation can happen in an osteoporotic bone or due to frequent entry of K-wire at the same entry point or thermal necrosis from high-speed thick wire drilling, or inadequate purchase at the far cortex, or inappropriate placement of K-wire in soft tissues, and not in the bone, which is a technical error. Sometimes the wire can get pulled out while doing a dressing or can get caught in clothes or bedspreads. It is to be noted that K-wire

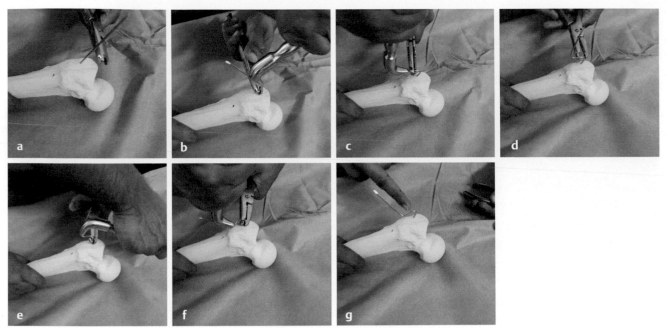

Fig. 1.15 (a–g) Technique of bending K-wire as close as 180 degrees demonstrated step-by-step on above model.

fixation is a flimsy fixation and that patient needs to be educated to take care and not to give undue load, which can lead to the loss of fixation. Loosening and pulling out of K-wire is common in the head of humerus fractures, especially from second week onward. Hence, in anticipation one can add more number of K-wires to fix the fracture so that if one or two fail, the others will still hold. (Pin loosening and back out in 2 weeks postop: additional two more K-wires in an osteoporotic bone could have been a better choice.) It is not uncommon to have K-wire misplaced outside the bone, which is a technical error leading to the loss of fixation. **Table 1.2** gives the reasons for loss of fixation (**Fig. 1.16**).

Most important of all is that the surgeon has the proprioception and feel of how good the fixation is and if not happy it is better to redo rather than accept a flimsy fixation which will give way in the immediate postoperative period.

Loss of Reduction

Losing the reduction is a serious issue and the reasons are similar to loss of fixation as discussed previously. Early pullout of the wire or inadvertent force through this precarious fixation can be a cause. Sometimes the fixation of the fracture may not neutralize all the forces

Table 1.2 Reasons for loss of fixation

- Not a bicortical fixation
- Far cortex purchase close to the fracture
- Convergence of all K-wires at one point in the far cortex purchase
- Too many times poking in and out of the same track
- Don't overshoot the tip beyond the far cortex fixation as reversing or pulling out the wire will cause loosening
- K-wire rotating freely while bending the wire
- Osteoporotic bone with flimsy hold where additional K-wires may be necessary
- Smooth pins have less pullout strength than threaded pins

of deformation as the K-wire fixation is not ideally positioned according to the personality of the fracture. It can also happen due to the fixation too close to the fracture which can give way or the wire may get bent.

Migration of K-Wire

Migration of K-wire is an unwanted complication and is more disastrous in humerus and clavicle fractures in which it can migrate into the chest. The K-wire should be bent adequately so that it does not migrate beyond the

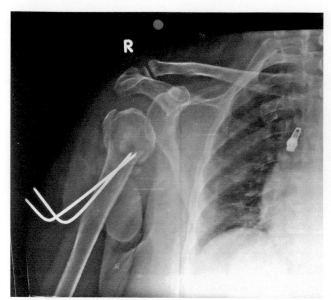

Fig. 1.16 Loss of fixation in proximal humerus fracture due to back out of K-wires.

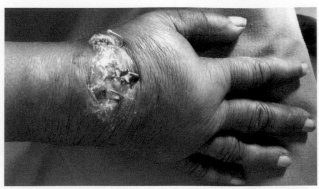

Fig. 1.17 Pin tract infection with surrounding erythema.

near cortex whether buried or outside the skin. Threaded K-wires are used for this purpose in the humerus for better purchase and for preventing migration. However, while removing this threaded K-wire in surgery, one must rotate anticlockwise rather than pulling hard causing pain for the patient. Regular periodic X-rays are mandatory to prevent pin breakage and migration. The unburied K-wire getting buried under the skin is also a problem. One can overcome this by cutting the K-wire at least 2 cm away from the bend. Use of a paraffin gauze dressing around the wire can prevent the migration to some extent. Migrating wire indicates loss of fixation and that wire needs to be removed at the earliest.

Breakage of K-Wire

Breakage of K-wire is a rare event. Intraoperatively this can happen while the surgeon exerts undesirable bending force while drilling for long duration. Again this is possible when K-wire comes into contact with another metal or another K-wire that does not allow advancement of the wire. The broken K-wire can be removed under fluoroscopy guidance, in case if the broken tip is extramedullary. In case of intramedullary breakage, one can attempt removal of the broken wire by over drilling the entry point, thereby facilitating the use of a straight mosquito forceps or small disc punch to remove the remnant wire. However, this results in excessive soft tissue

trauma and compromise of distal fragment bone stock. Another alternative method is to angulate the extremity to open the fracture site. A percutaneous incision can then be made to reach the opened-out cortex to facilitate passing a mosquito forceps to hold the wire to push it out through the entry hole.

Patients with joint transfixation K-wires, for example, distal radioulnar joint transfixation for distal radioulnar joint instability or humeroulnar K-wiring, will require additional above-elbow cast to prevent movement and breakage of wire. Intra-articular wire migration may require arthroscopy for removal.

Pin Tract Infection

Pin tract infection is a known complication but can be minimized by assessing the risk factors. Patients with diabetes and those with skin diseases are prone to infection. K-wire at the site of immobilization rarely results in infection like supracondylar fracture K-wiring immobilized with above-elbow plaster of Paris (POP) slab. The infection can vary from minor pin tract infection to severe form of osteomyelitis. Movement of soft tissues around the wire or a loose K-wire is a predisposing factor for infection. Inadequate soft tissue release around K-wire results in collection of sebum underneath with scab over it acting as a nidus for bacterial growth. Adequate skin and soft tissue release is necessary to prevent this problem. Maintenance of pin site by removing the scab and moving the skin in two different directions (length and breadthwise) to prevent skin adhesion to K-wire and blockage of exudate is important (**Fig. 1.17**). Tips to avoid pin tract infection are mentioned in **Table 1.3.**

Table 1.3 Tips to avoid pin tract infection

- After skin incision, artery forceps must be used first to separate the soft tissue and then K-wire should be passed
- K-wire painted with betadine (povidone iodine)
- Slow speed drilling to prevent thermal necrosis
- Avoid too many pricks
- No skin tethering
- Loose pins to be removed

Skin Tethering

Skin tethering occurs due to technical inadequacy. This problem can be prevented either by starting with skin incision followed by using artery forceps to spread the tissues apart and to reach the bone, or by making liberal skin and soft tissue release at the point of entry of K-wire through the skin. Adjacent joints are moved fully to assess for any restriction of movements and for tethering of skin (**Fig. 1.18a, b**). Adequate skin and soft tissue release will prevent pain, infection, and stiffness.

Stiffness

The patient usually returns with a complaint that "something is not right." It can be of various etiology, ranging from K-wire causing skin tethering, soft tissue impalement, infection, inadequate improper fixation causing pain, tip of the K-wire irritating the joint surface or soft tissues, transfixation of the joint, inadequate physiotherapy, inadequate fracture reduction with fracture ends tethering the soft tissues, prolonged period of immobilization, reflex sympathetic dystrophy, and personality disorders. The chondral damage in joint transfixation is of only theoretical risk but practically nil.

Physeal Damage and Growth Arrest

Transphyseal smooth K-wires for fixing pediatric fractures/dislocations is the safest implant across the physis even today. Even though there is a theoretical disadvantage of damaging the physis, the damage is so negligible that practically it is of no significance. It is very safe to use, provided a gentle and apt fixation is done without multiple attempts. The only detrimental effect is

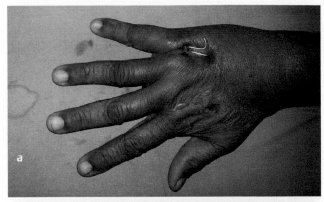
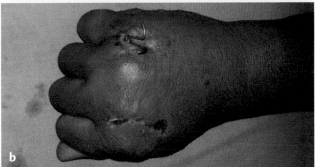

Fig. 1.18 (a, b) Skin puckering with limitation of flexion at metacarpophalangeal joint.

pin tract infection and if it is severe can lead on to osteomyelitis and physeal damage. Scrupulous treatment of early infection is recommended with antibiotics and early pin removal to avoid this complication.

Future Perspectives

K-wires with various coatings aimed at reducing the infection rate, either in the form of a coating to resist infection (monolaurin-coated K-wires, tobramycin–PDLLA (poly-DL-lactide) coated titanium Kirschner-wire, antimicrobial silver multilayer coating) or elute antibiotics (nanofiber composite-coating technology), over a period of time are in experimental stage. Other coatings such as nanostructured hydroxyapatite-coated wires have proven satisfactory results in lab results, enhancing bone formation around the wires. However, these special coatings are still in laboratory evaluation and require further validation to look for any adverse effects and their cost-effectiveness and may be considered for use in selected patients such as uncontrolled diabetes, patients on chronic steroid therapy, and poor skin condition.

Conclusion

K-wire is an inevitable, simple, cost-effective device freely available on the shelves of orthopedic operating theaters used in day-to-day practice by common orthopedic surgeons and hand and plastic surgeons not only for fracture management, but also as an instrument of multifarious nature. K-wires are an immensely useful implant in the current clinical scenario, which has stood the test of time. They are "designed to last and be around forever."

2 Hand

General Principles

K-wiring is the most common method of implant fixation for fractures of small bones of the hand. Stiffness, pain, and deformity are the major concerns in treating this fracture. Though some patients are unfortunate to have poor outcome due to the nature of the injury, poor outcome may be due to poor technique of fixation as seen in **Figs. 2.1** and **2.2a, b**. In some patients, poor outcome may occur despite good looking X-rays and this may be due to poor soft tissue handling or wrong selection of patient or poor compliance with hand physiotherapy care.

Again a good looking radiograph may not guarantee a good functional outcome especially in the hand. If the surgery is not done properly respecting the soft tissues, stiffness is an invariable consequence. **Fig. 2.3a–d** shows the middle finger was stiff and straight impairing the functioning of the hand. The K-wire has been passed in different directions impaling the extensor expansion (oblique retinacular ligament) at proximal interphalangeal joint (PIPJ) level and possibly the collateral ligament. In this case, the patient was not able to actively flex the finger from day 1 postoperative period because

of extensor tendon tethering, which led on to tightness. One should understand the anatomy of safe corridors to insert the K-wire to start active range of motion exercises at the earliest.

There is a lacuna in the literature on standard technique to be adopted or the principle to be followed on K-wiring hand fractures. We have made an attempt to perform a desirable way of K-wire fixation in order to get the best clinical outcome with an "on-table active examination test" to check for full active finger movements and to rule out soft tissue tethering, as most of the times these procedures are done using digital or wrist block anesthesia. We always show to the patient the complete range of movement done by him/her in the operating room; this boosts up his/her confidence to work on postoperative physiotherapy to achieve the same.

The safe corridor for entry of K-wire in finger has been mapped for proper understanding and execution of the procedure. The indications for K-wiring include unstable fractures, open fractures, avulsion fractures (e.g., central slip avulsion, mallet finger), and failed conservative treatment.

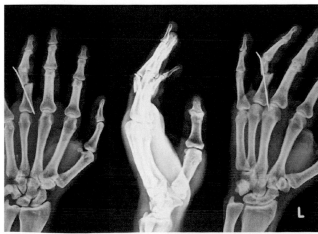

Fig. 2.1 K-wire was not holding the distal fragment and fracture was malaligned.

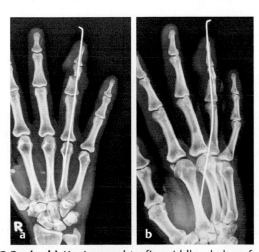

Fig. 2.2 **(a, b)** K-wire used to fix middle phalanx fracture has overshot proximally and impaled the volar soft tissues.

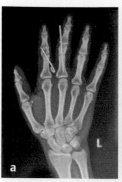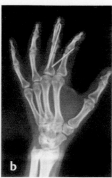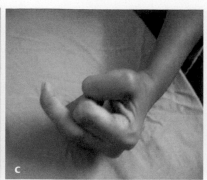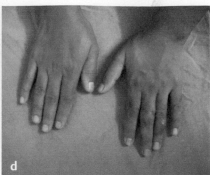

Fig. 2.3 **(a–d)** K-wire not passed through safe portal resulting in stiff finger.

Indications of K-Wiring of Phalangeal and Metacarpal Fractures

- Unstable fractures.
- Fractures with rotation, angular deformity, and shortening.
- Multiple phalangeal fractures in the same hand.
- Open fractures.
- Avulsion fractures.
- Failed conservative treatment.

The advantage of K-wire fixation in hand is achieving stable fixation for early mobilization. The patient must be motivated for immediate postoperative range of movement exercises for good clinical outcome. In closed hand fractures, K-wire is generally removed in 3 to 4 weeks' time when the fracture is sticky enough. One need not wait for radiological evidence of callus formation for the removal of wire as this may result in stiffness. There are few exemptions such as open fractures or severely comminuted fracture with significant soft tissue damage or avulsion fractures in which we delay the removal of K-wire.

Safe Corridor in a Finger

The safe corridor in a finger is an area where a K-wire can be passed with minimal soft tissues trauma and without impaling major soft tissue structures such as extensor expansion, neurovascular structure, and flexor tendons, thus allowing relatively pain-free active range of movements and preventing stiffness.

We did a cadaveric study in hand and passed multiple K-wires in each phalanx by visually identifying the extensor expansion and mapped the safe portal avoiding any tethering of the same. This is further tested by manual pulling of flexor and extensor tendons for full passive flexion and extension of fingers so that there is no restriction of movements (**Fig. 2.4a, b**). Mapping was done in each phalanx both in flexion and extension of the fingers and the safe corridor was identified.

Proximal Phalanx

A triangular wide area of safe zone is present dorsolaterally and dorsomedially on either side of the extensor tendon in the base of the proximal phalanx (PPX).

The PPX shaft is a dangerous zone; it has extensor expansion all around the lateral side (lumbrical and interossei tendon) and neurovascular structures, and flexor tendons on the volar side.

In the PPX head, dorsomedial and dorsolateral small triangular area is safe in flexion and this corridor gets obliterated in extension.

Middle Phalanx

In the base of the middle phalanx (MPX), there is a small triangular safe corridor in flexion of the PIPJ dorsomedially and dorsolaterally, between the central slip and lateral band. Shaft of the MPX is usually a dangerous area to pass the K-wires, as the lateral band and oblique retinacular ligament pass across the lateral aspect. The head of MPX has a wide safe zone dorsomedially and dorsolaterally in both flexion and extension.

Distal Phalanx

In the distal phalanx (DPX) the tip is safe, and the dangerous zones are dorsal and volar insertion points of long extensor and flexor tendon, respectively (**Fig. 2.5a, b**).

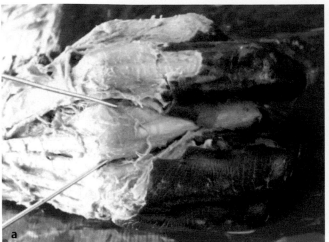

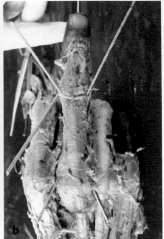

Fig. 2.4 (a, b) A cadaveric study demonstrating K-wires passed through safe corridor in phalanges.

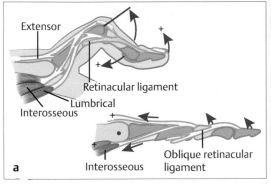

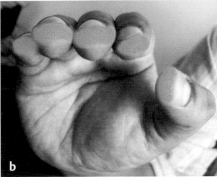

Fig. 2.5 (a, b) Mapping of safe corridor in flexion and extension of the finger and at finger tips.

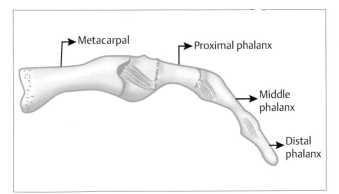

Fig. 2.6 Eccentric insertion of the collateral ligaments.

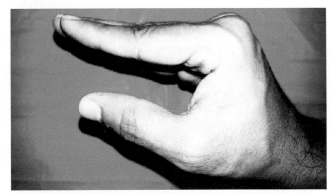

Fig. 2.7 Safe position of the hand (James position).

The K-wires are never inserted from volar surface of the finger as it is a dangerous zone because of the presence of flexor tendons and its sheath.

Safe Position of Hand (Intrinsic Plus Hand)

The position of immobilization should be the one that leads to the least amount of stiffness and early functional recovery of the joint. In the hand the metacarpophalangeal joints (MCPJs) are flexed to 70 degrees, PIPJ and distal interphalangeal joints (DIPJs) are in full extension, thumb is in abduction such that the collateral ligaments are at maximum stretched position in this posture, and the wrist is in 30-degree dorsiflexion (**Figs. 2.6** and **2.7**).

In exceptional situations in which the K-wire could not be passed through the safe corridor, it could be inserted in any port of desired entry for the fracture pattern with least tethering by holding the fingers in functional position. These K-wires should be removed at the earliest as soon as the fracture is sticky enough and stable. Avulsion fracture (bony mallet finger, central slip avulsion fracture) is an exemption from safe corridor entry, where there is a direct or indirect reduction of the fracture with K-wire stabilization (**Fig. 2.8**).

Partial Intra-Articular Fracture

Partial Intra-Articular Fracture without Joint Dislocation or Subluxation

In DIPJ (bony mallet), PIPJ (volar plate avulsion, central slip avulsion fracture), MCPJ, and carpometacarpal joint (CMCJ), intra-articular fracture, unicondylar fracture of the PPX head, or MPX fracture can be treated by direct K-wire fixation method that are discussed under each section giving importance to the fracture fragment.

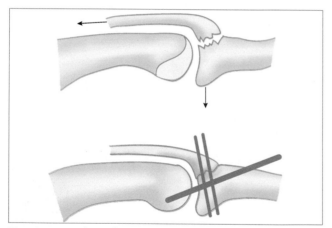

Fig. 2.8 Avulsion fracture with direct transfixation K-wire and force neutralization K-wire to transfix the joint and immobilize.

Partial Intra-Articular Fracture with Joint Subluxation

If there is an associated joint subluxation or dislocation in partial intra-articular fracture (either because the articular fragment size is >40% of total articular surface attributing to joint instability or the associated capsule and ligamentous injuries causing joint subluxation), primary importance is given to joint reduction and congruency of joint surface by K-wire transfixation, for example, condylar fracture head of the PPX or MPX with joint subluxation, mallet finger dislocation, fracture dislocation at the PPX base, Bennett fracture dislocation, etc. This transfixation across the joint can be intramedullary transfixation or a cross K-wire transfixation across the reduced joint. This may bring the fracture fragment back to the place (indirect reduction). **Table 2.1** states general rule of thumb in K-wiring phalanges and metacarpals.

Ligamentotaxis Using Single K-Wire[1]

It is a case of innovative method of treating comminuted intra- and extra-articular phalanx fracture. Treating comminuted phalangeal fracture is a challenge faced by orthopedic surgeons worldwide. Fractures of phalanges are the most common upper limb bony injuries. The difficulties in treating phalangeal injuries of hand is to design intervention protocols that recognize the need to maintain fracture stability for maximal bone healing, while also introducing early, controlled motion protocols to preserve soft tissue integrity. Ligamentotaxis involves molding fracture fragments into alignment by applying tension across the fracture using surrounding intact soft tissue envelope. The traction and the countertraction

Table 2.1   General rule of thumb in K-wiring phalanges and metacarpals

Proximal phalanx fractures	Antegrade double intramedullary K-wire from the dorsomedial and dorsolateral safe corridor entry
Middle phalanx fractures	Retrograde joint transfixation intramedullary K-wire from distal phalanx tip to the middle phalanx; rarely K-wire from dorsomedial or dorsolateral head of middle phalanx
Distal phalanx fractures	Retrograde intramedullary K-wire from the tip of distal phalanx
Metacarpal shaft and base	Retrograde intramedullary K-wire from the metacarpal head
Metacarpal neck and head fractures	Antegrade prebent intramedullary K-wire with eccentric insertion from the metacarpal base with few exemptions

[1]Rex C, Patel K, Sandeep KM. A method of treating comminuted phalangeal fractures by ligamentotaxis using a single Kirschner wire. J Hand Surg Eur Vol. 2017;42(9):971-972.

restore the length and guide alignment of the fracture fragments, which are otherwise difficult to control. External fixation both static and dynamic is an effective method of treatment particularly when internal fixation is not possible due to comminution and associated soft tissue injury. Routinely ligamentotaxis was done using miniexternal fixator for phalanx; we describe a novel method for ligamentotaxis of phalanx using single smooth K-wire of suitable diameter as an unlocked intramedullary nail, achieving and maintaining fracture reduction. This is a simple, minimally invasive technique with good patient compliance and excellent functional outcome.

Indications and Inclusion Criteria

- Displaced intra-articular fractures of phalanges.
- Comminuted extra-articular fractures of phalanges.
- Fracture subluxation/dislocation of IPJ/CMCJ.
- Fractures less than 1-week-old.
- Closed and open fracture phalanx.

Surgical Procedure

Fracture was reduced by traction and countertraction maneuver, and with the fluoroscopic guidance the fracture reduction was confirmed. Straight intramedullary K-wire was passed from distal tip of the finger crossing the fracture, maintaining the reduction with traction, and stabilizing the fracture. The size (diameter) of the K-wire is determined by the narrowest part of the phalanx that is crossed during insertion. It is necessary to use the thickest possible wire that can cross through the isthmus of medullary canal for a snug fix. The K-wire was placed subchondrally to maintain distraction at fracture site. Being a non-weight-bearing bone, the distraction is easily maintained by the firm purchase of the K-wire tip in the hard bone (subchondral area). The neutralization of forces from extensor and flexor tendon due to immobilization in extension does not allow collapse from extrinsic loading. The thickness of K-wire is important for a firm intramedullary snug fix. The parking of K-wire subchondrally can be at the base of phalanx or at the head of adjacent phalanx. Adjacent joint mobilization was started immediately. With the functional position

of the hand being interphalangeal joints in extension (James position), transfixation with K-wire in extension does not lead onto stiffness after early removal as the collateral ligaments are in maximum stretched position. Normally K-wire is removed at the end of 3 to 4 weeks depending upon comminution and soft tissue damage.

Salient Features of Introduction of Single K-Wire for Distraction Ligamentotaxis

- The thickness of K-wire must correspond to the narrowest part of medullary canal of the phalanx it crosses, and it is usually the DPX that determines the size. The suitable thickness of K-wire passed from DPX tip is determined by the isthmus of medullary canal of DPX (**Fig. 2.9a, b**). Compared to thin K-wire in the first picture, the thicker K-wire in the second picture matches the isthmus of DPX for a snug fix.
- Going past the fracture site, one should maintain the traction in distraction mode by checking in C-arm before parking in the subchondral bone (**Fig. 2.10a–c**). The K-wire entering the hard subchondral bone of PPX head causes distraction (increase in joint space) at PIPJ and this force is lost as soon as it enters the hollow medullary canal resulting in collapse at PIPJ (**Fig. 2.11a, b**).
- In case of comminuted fracture shaft phalanx with adequate proximal segment, one may park the

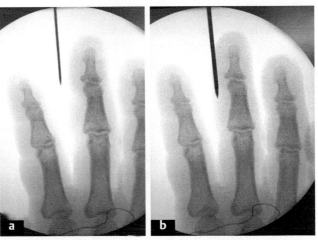

Fig. 2.9 (a, b) To assess the diameter of the isthmus of the distal phalanx (DPX) and the corresponding thickness of K-wire.

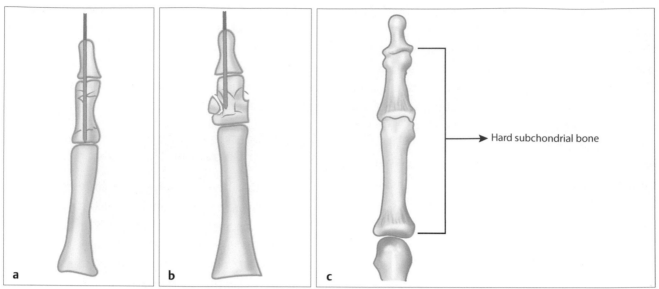

Fig. 2.10 (a) K-wire entering the medullary canal of collapsed middle phalanx (MPX). (b) Parking the tip of K-wire at subchondral base of middle phalanx (MPX) in distraction mode. (c) Hard subchondral bone on either sides of interphalangeal (IP) and metacarpophalangeal (MCP) joints.

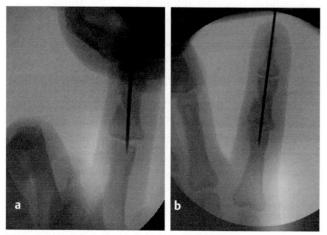

Fig. 2.11 (a) Demonstration of distraction at proximal interphalangeal (PIP) joint on entering the hard subchondral bone of proximal phalanx (PPX) head. (b) Wire passing the subchondral area and entering the medullary canal of PPX results in collapse of the PIP joint.

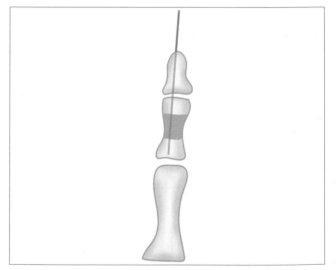

Fig. 2.12 In comminuted shaft fracture of middle phalanx (MPX) K-wire tip can be parked at the base of the middle phalanx.

K-wire tip in the base of the same phalanx at the subchondral bone (**Fig. 2.12**).

- Fracture extending to the base of the phalanx or intra-articular comminution requires transfixation across the joint to the head of the phalanx proximal to it (**Fig. 2.13**).
- In case if one goes past the head, the tip of K-wire can be taken to the subchondral bone at the base of PPX (**Fig. 2.14**).

- Working length is between the isthmus and the tip of K-wire in the hard subchondral bone (**Fig. 2.15**).
- Too much distraction can happen in severe soft tissue injury or bone loss where one can telescope forcefully the distal segment to the desired level. Too much distraction due to soft tissue damage is dangerous as it can jeopardize the circulation. One must always check on the vascularity of the fingertip at the end of the procedure.

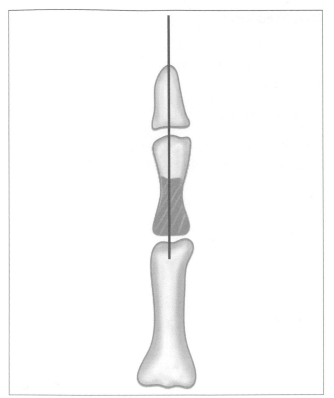

Fig. 2.13   Comminuted intra-articular extension of middle phalanx (MPX) needs parking at proximal phalanx (PPX) head.

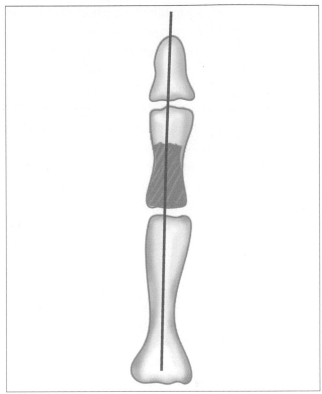

Fig. 2.14   Accidentally if the K-wire tip has crossed beyond the hard subchondral bone of proximal phalanx (PPX) head, it can be parked at the base of PPX in distraction mode.

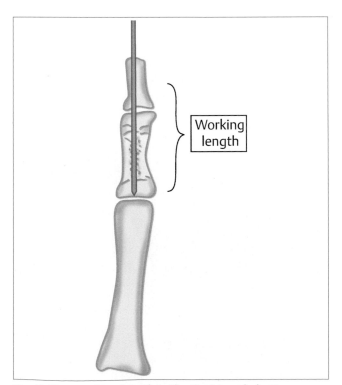

Fig. 2.15   Working length in the K-wiring phalanx.

Management of comminuted shaft phalanx fractures with shortening and intra-articular fractures with subluxation/dislocation has always posed a challenge to the orthopedic surgeon in terms of reduction of fracture, maintenance of reduction while the fracture is healing, and the mobility of the joints during and after the fracture union. Although several methods are used in the treatment of intra-articular phalangeal fractures, there is no universally accepted ideal method. The joint stiffness, deformity, and degenerative osteoarthritis remain as significant complications. Postunion functioning of the joint is the most difficult part of the management of the comminuted intra/juxta-articular fractures because of stiffness and pain. Patient's expectations are very high and good results are not always possible due to severity of injury, soft tissue damage, and the periarticular fibrosis/tendon tethering that result in the process of healing.

Ligamentotaxis using single K-wire is an innovative method that can be used by any orthopedic surgeon with minimal resources and minimal expertise. Routine use of mini-external fixator for ligamentotaxis is sidelined by the usage of this K-wiring technique. External fixator has many disadvantages like pin-tract infection, tethering of soft tissue, unfriendly to the patient, difficulty in technicality for achieving a three-dimensional reduction, and gross stiffness. External fixator requires longer time to maintain the length and usually produces reasonable radiological outcome with poor functional outcome. Pain scale during the period of fixation and removal of external fixator definitely far exceeds than this method of minimally invasive K-wire fixation with little pain. Again soft tissue plastic procedures are easily done unlike external fixator treatment which compromises the treatment and outcome.

Pin-tract infection was not reported in our series of 48 patients and if in case it arises it is a minor problem which can be taken care easily. Being a joint spanning K-wire and placed for 3 to 4 weeks, the general apprehension is joint stiffness or damage to the joint surface. In our study this temporary joint stiffness eased up quickly with physiotherapy after K-wire removal and by 6 to 8 weeks all regained almost full functional range of motion. It is more of theoretical apprehension; practically it does not affect the function. Moreover the surface area of the cartilage injured by a K-wire through a joint is less than 5% which is insignificant to cause a potential serious damage. Some residual stiffness in two patients in comparison to normal was due to tethering of the extensor tendon in a comminuted fracture resulting in limitation of finger movements, and/or the fracture pattern itself, and/or the patient's little effort in rehabilitation. No loss of reduction or shortening was found on comparing the first and last X-rays.

This technique can be easily mastered by all orthopedic surgeons for excellent patient outcome. It not only obviates the need of complex open reduction and internal fixation or an uncomfortable external fixator, but also gives better functional results.

Single K-wire ligamentotaxis using the method described is ideally suited for comminuted extra-articular and intra-articular phalanx fractures. It is a simple, reliable, less expensive, and reproducible technique with less operative time and proven good functional outcome.

Case Scenario 1

Comminuted fracture PPX with angulation and shortening treated with single K-wire ligamentotaxis (**Fig. 2.16a, b**).

Case Scenario 2

Intra-articular fracture subluxation of MPX treated with single K-wire ligamentotaxis (**Fig. 2.17a–d**).

Case Scenario 3

Fracture dislocation of PIPJ treated with single K-wire ligamentotaxis (**Fig. 2.18a–c**).

Case Scenario 4

Restoration of length and alignment of MPX and DPX fractures of F4 and F5 (**Fig. 2.19a–d**).

In an intra-articular fracture of IPJ, direct fragment-specific fixation for perfect articular alignment and reduction of the joint or indirect joint stabilization method is an ideal choice.

In a situation where the articular fragments are too comminuted for fixation or the intra-articular fracture leads on to joint instability in the form of subluxation or dislocation or multiple comminuted phalanx fracture in the same finger may warrant single intramedullary K-wire technique using ligamentotaxis principle. The other option would be an external fixator in dynamic mode or closed traction techniques.

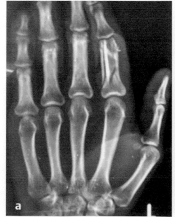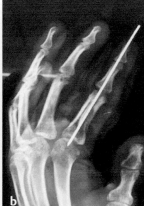

Fig. 2.16 (a, b) Comminuted proximal phalanx (PPX) treated with ligamentotaxis principle by parking tip of K-wire in metacarpal head in functional flexion position.

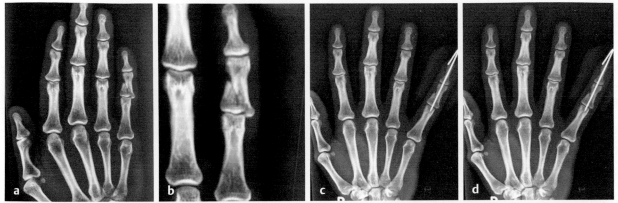

Fig. 2.17 (a–d) Fracture subluxation of proximal interphalangeal joint (PIPJ) reduced and treated with single intramedullary K-wire in distraction mode.

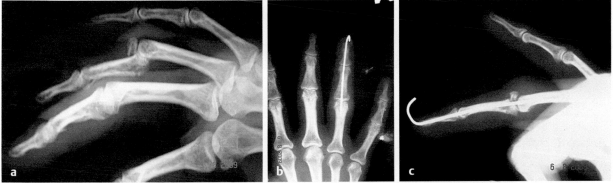

Fig. 2.18 (a–c) Fracture dislocation of proximal interphalangeal joint (PIPJ) reduced and fixed with single intramedullary K-wire in distraction mode.

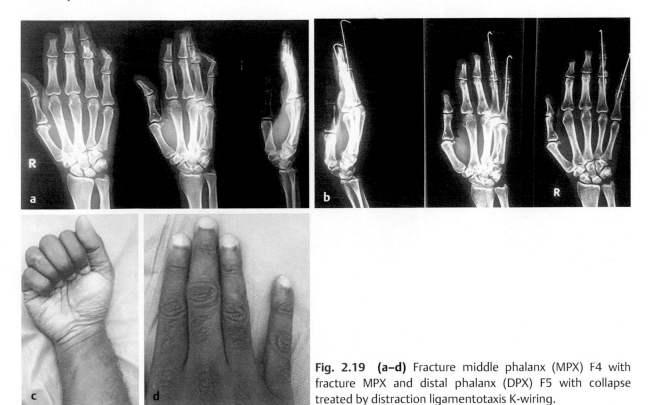

Fig. 2.19 (a–d) Fracture middle phalanx (MPX) F4 with fracture MPX and distal phalanx (DPX) F5 with collapse treated by distraction ligamentotaxis K-wiring.

Distal Phalanx

Bony Mallet Avulsion Fracture Base of Distal Phalanx

Case Scenario 1

The extensor tendon avulsed fragment was manipulated and reduced using a 18-gauge hypodermic needle and maintained in extension. An intramedullary K-wire was passed from the DPX tip through IPJ to PPX in 0-degree extension. A direct K-wire transfixing the avulsion fragment of extensor tendon was also inserted in the base of DPX. If the fragment is too small and displaced, a pull-out suture can be done by open method.

The joint transfixation K-wire was maintained for a period of 6 weeks and fragment-specific direct K-wire fixation was removed at 4 weeks. Mallet finger night splint was used for a period of 6 months (**Fig. 2.20a–g**).

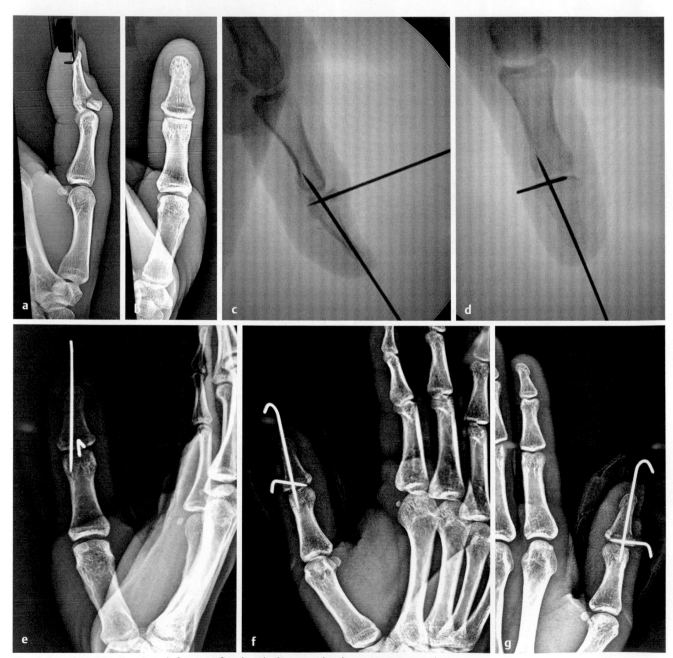

Fig. 2.20 **(a–g)** Mallet thumb fracture fixed with direct and indirect K-wiring technique.

Case Scenario 2

Here the avulsed fragment was large and rotated. It was not amenable for a perfect closed reduction. Hence an open reduction was necessary to derotate and reduce the avulsed fragment on the bed anatomically. One direct K-wire to transfix was inserted to one side of the fragment so that it does not hinder the placement of central joint transfixation intramedullary K-wire across DIPJ. Once these two wires were used to hold directly and indirectly the fracture reduction yet another third K-wire was inserted from the dorsum directly transfixing the huge avulsed fragment for additional stability and to prevent tilting. The fragment-specific K-wires were removed at the end of 4 weeks and joint transfixation K-wire was removed at the end of 6 weeks (**Fig. 2.21a–e**).

Swan Neck Deformity Secondary to Mallet Finger (Fig. 2.22a–h)

A chronic longstanding malunited bony mallet avulsion fracture will result in secondary swan neck deformity. As the deformity was flexible, a soft tissue balancing procedure was done. The hyperextended PIPJ was kept in 20-degree flexion and a joint transfixation cross K-wiring was done. The DIPJ was fixed in neutral position by central intramedullary K-wire from DPX tip to the MPX. The extensor digitorum tendon insertion to DPX was erased; the bony spur was excised and a pull-out stitch of the tendon through DPX base was anchored to a button on the pulp of the fingertip with adequate tension. All the wires were removed at the end of 6 weeks and then a mallet finger night splint was continued for a period of 6 months. Good final correction was obtained at the end of 6 months postsurgery (**Fig. 2.22a–h**).

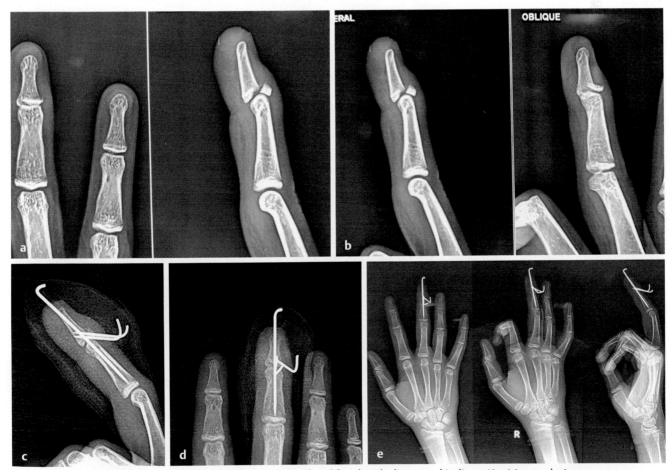

Fig. 2.21 (a–e) Mallet finger with subluxation corrected and fixed with direct and indirect K-wiring technique.

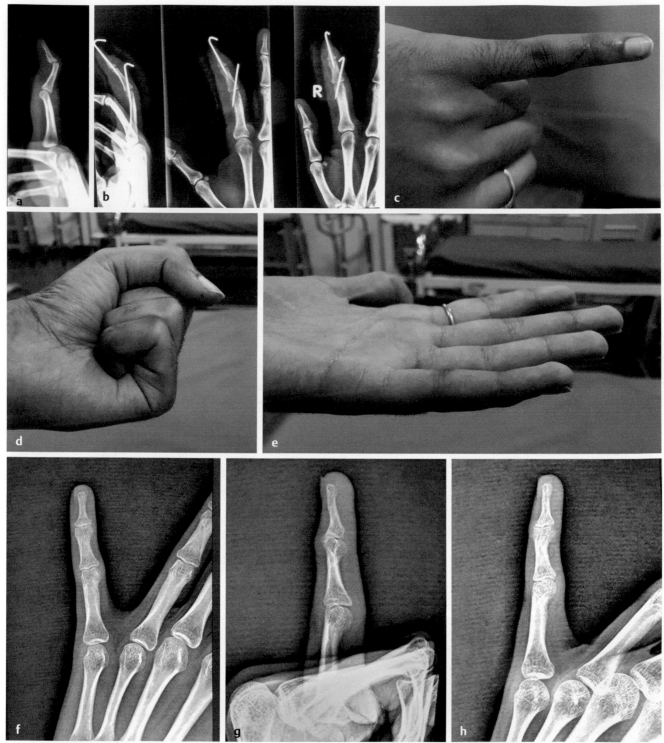

Fig. 2.22 **(a–h)** Flexible swan neck deformity due to Mallet finger was corrected by soft tissue balancing and correction maintained with joint transfixation K-wire in different manners (intramedullary for distal interphalangeal joint [DIPJ] and cross K-wire for proximal interphalangeal joint [PIPJ]) with functional results.

Distal Phalanx Fracture in Little Finger

DPX fracture at the waist level leads to flexion of the distal fragment and extension of its base, which is caused by the extensor expansion insertion (**Fig. 2.23a, b**). This causes nail bed disruption and cosmetically scarred nail permanently if left alone to heal. To prevent this, one must anatomically reduce the fracture for perfect matching of nail bed. A retrograde K-wiring with the entry point centered on the DPX tip in anteroposterior (AP) view is identified. In lateral view the point of entry must be slightly dorsal and directed parallel to the dorsal cortex, thereby skirting the dorsal cortex for perfect reduction of the fracture. The method of reduction is shown in **Fig. 2.24.** (Once the fracture is transfixed anatomically with perfect nail bed matching, skin laceration rarely needs suturing because of good coaptation.)

At the point of entry one must spend some time for a perfect position of K-wire insertion by checking in C-arm image intensifier at different positions before advancing the K-wire intramedullary. Once a wrong tract is created, it is literally difficult to change the direction of K-wire again. There is only one chance to go and get the position corrected. Slow advancement without piercing the far cortex is very important, and 0.75-mm K-wires are used for this (**Fig. 2.25a–e**).

Thin K-wire is always preferred as it is desirable to change the direction; once a wrong passage is created using a thick K-wire, redirecting the K-wire becomes difficult.

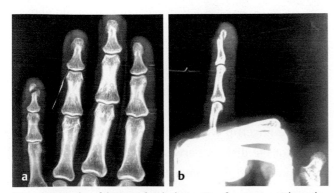

Fig. 2.23 (a, b) Distal phalanx tip fracture with volar displacement.

Open Distal Phalanx Fracture of Middle Finger with Closed Mallet Finger Deformity (Fig. 2.26a–f)

In this case, the DPX fracture was transfixed spanning across the DIPJ in extension for correction of mallet finger deformity. K-wiring was done in a retrograde manner and the wire was maintained for 6 weeks in mallet finger deformity correction. This was followed by mallet finger night splint which was given for another 6 weeks.

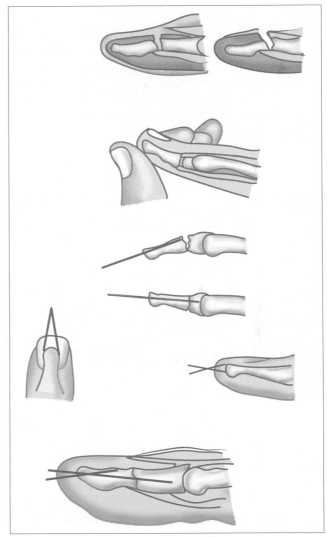

Fig. 2.24 Entry through the tip of phalanx is technically demanding and should be checked in both anteroposterior and lateral views before proceeding further, and usually it is just subungual and parallel to nail.

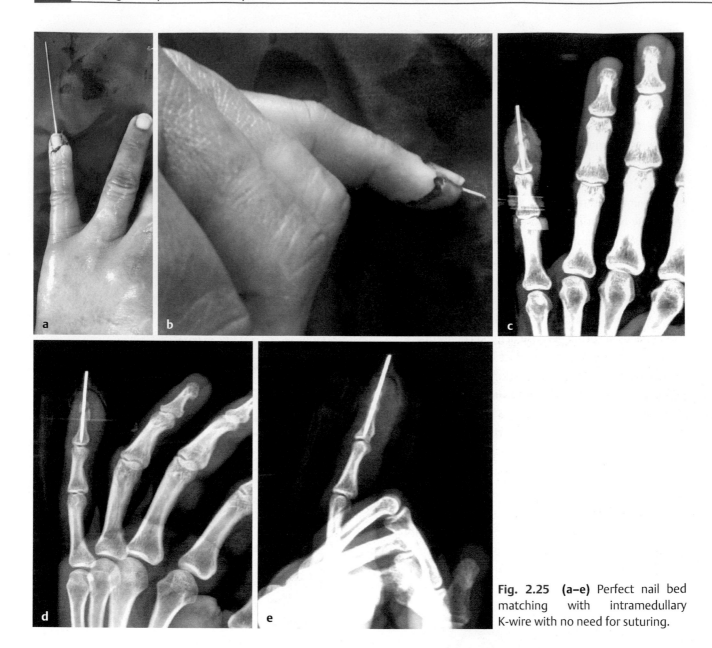

Fig. 2.25 (a–e) Perfect nail bed matching with intramedullary K-wire with no need for suturing.

Open Distal Phalanx Fracture with Nail Bed Laceration (Fig. 2.27a, b)

Subtotal amputation of the crushed fingertip hanging loose with minimal soft tissue attachment and was crushed. The vascularity of the tissue needs to be examined thoroughly. One should be careful while debriding the tissue, not to injure the intact digital artery. Under local anesthesia (plain lignocaine without adrenaline) gentle wash was provided with Savlon soap (Johnson & Johnson, New Brunswick, New Jersey) and Betadine (Purdue Products L.P., Stamford, Connecticut). Without

twisting or turning in retrograde manner, the K-wire was passed from fingertip intramedullary through the fracture site and into the proximal fragment. One should hold the fingertip while drilling to prevent a complete swivel of the digit; otherwise the digital artery will go into spasm and gangrene. Two stitches were done to secure the nail bed and skin.

This procedure can also be done by antegrade K-wiring through the fracture site in to the DPX tip exiting just under the nail and railroading in zig zag manner, back in to the proximal fragment. Anatomical reduction

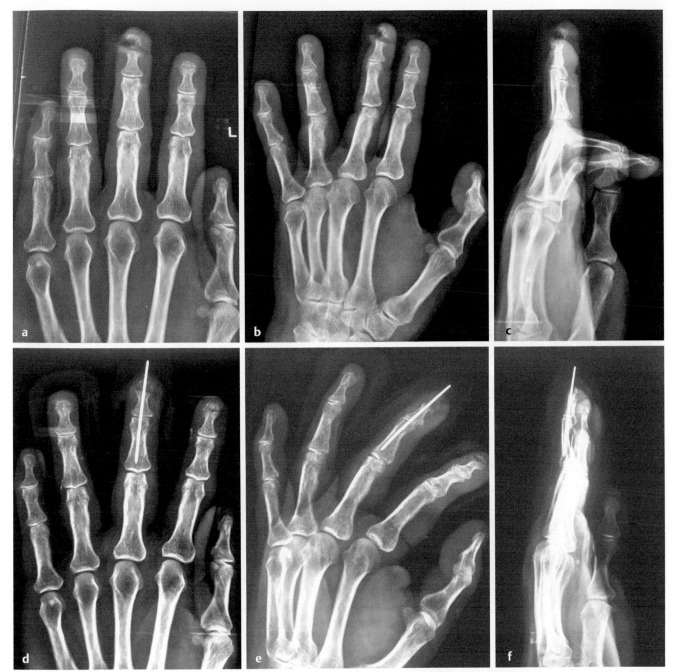

Fig. 2.26 (a–f) Open distal phalanx (DPX) fracture with open mallet deformity was treated with intramedullary K-wire transfixing the distal interphalangeal joint (DIPJ).

gives good approximation without any deformation of nail when it grows.

Displaced Distal Phalanx Shaft Fracture (Fig. 2.28a–f)

This fracture is commonly associated with nail bed injury and the distal fragment gets flexed and dorsally angulated. In a crush the nail gets avulsed from the bed and dorsal displacement of the fragment may jeopardize the cosmetic look of future nail growth. This deformity is corrected by selecting appropriate size K-wire considering the isthmus diameter in AP and lateral X-ray, and inserted from the tip of DPX parallel to the dorsal cortex. Keeping the fracture reduced, the wire is passed across

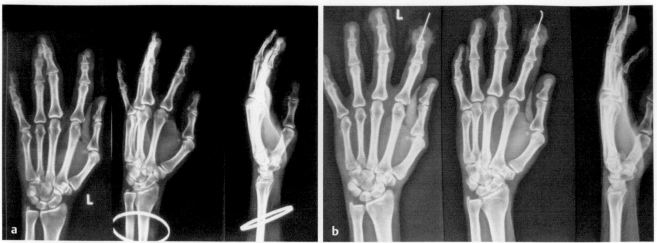

Fig. 2.27 **(a, b)** Intramedullary distal phalanx (DPX) K-wire to reposition the fingertip.

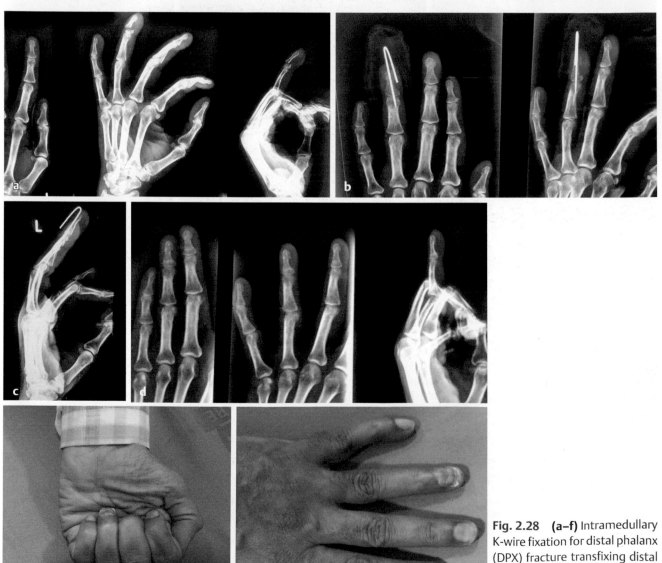

Fig. 2.28 **(a–f)** Intramedullary K-wire fixation for distal phalanx (DPX) fracture transfixing distal interphalangeal joint (DIPJ) for stability.

the base and through the DIPJ for better stability. The final result is obtained at the end of 6 weeks with good consolidation of fracture and good mobility.

Physeal Separation of Distal Phalanx

Index Finger

In a child with DPX physeal separation at the base following a sport injury, the DPX was extended and displaced with volar angulation. A 0.8-mm K-wire was used from the tip of the DPX entering intramedullary. The wire was used as a joystick to manipulate and reduce the DPX on to the epiphysis and transfixed as shown in good position (**Fig. 2.29a–f**).

Ring Finger

Type 1 puncture compound physeal fracture of DPX with separation of ring finger was reduced by closed means. The reduction was maintained with central intramedullary K-wire from fingertip to DIPJ and parking at the head of MPX. This wire was maintained for a period of 3 weeks and then removed. Further mobilization of the finger was done (**Fig. 2.30a–f**).

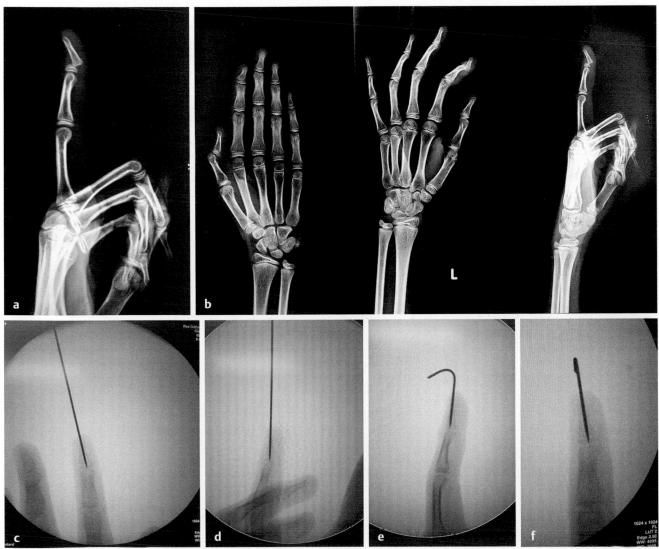

Fig. 2.29 (a–f) Physeal separation of distal phalanx (DPX) reduced and fixed with intramedullary K-wire from DPX tip to epiphysis.

Distal Interphalangeal Joint

Fusion of Interphalangeal Joint

Case Scenario 1

It is a case of distal interphalangeal joint fusion of middle finger. A 7-year-postmallet finger deformity with arthritic changes and pain was treated with deformity correction and arthrodesis of DIPJ. By open reduction and denuding the cartilage, the deformity was corrected at DIPJ. DIPJ was fused in 0-degree extension by passing an intramedullary 0.8-mm K-wire from the DPX tip to MPX.

The compression at the arthrodesis site was achieved by axial compression by the surgeon and maintenance by two cross K-wires, which finally looks like a trident. These wires are maintained for at least 10 to 12 weeks until the radiological evidence of fusion (**Fig. 2.31a–f**).

Case Scenario 2

It is a case of old unreduced rotary subluxation of interphalangeal joint thumb with secondary osteoarthritis with IPJ fusion thumb (**Fig. 2.32a–e**). After open reduction and denuding the articular surface, bleeding subchondral bone was exposed and good contact was established. Interphalangeal joint fusion was done in

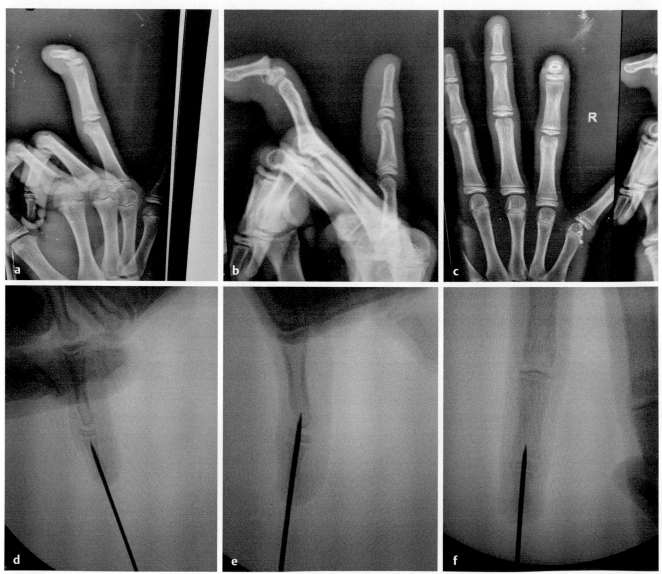

Fig. 2.30 **(a–f)** Distal phalanx (DPX) physeal seperation reduced and fixed with distal interphalangeal joint (DIPJ) transfixation intramedullary K-wire.

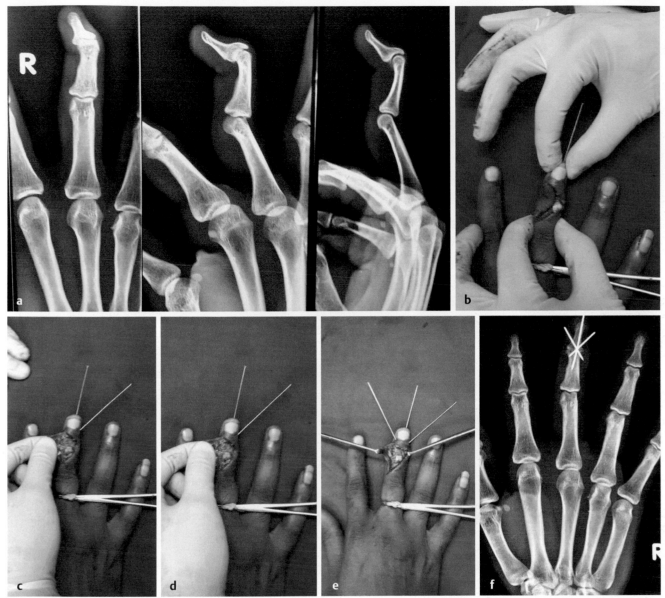

Fig. 2.31   (a–f) Distal interphalangeal joint (DIPJ) arthritis due to old malunited avulsion finger. Central intramedullary K-wire through the distal phalanx (DPX) and middle phalanx (MPX) passed after denuding the cartilage. The DIPJ cross K-wires were passed as shown by compressing.

extension using three K-wires. First, intramedullary K-wire was passed in a retrograde railroading zig zag technique and then cross K-wire was inserted with axial compression for a good rotational control.

Interphalangeal Joint Dislocation

Case Scenario 1

Interphalangeal joint dislocation thumb. X-ray shows the dorsal dislocation of the interphalangeal joint along with small volar chip avulsion fragment of thumb. Here after closed reduction the active flexion of IPJ was tested to rule out flexor pollicis longus avulsion. The flexor was working and the fragment was confirmed to be volar plate capsular avulsion fracture.

Because of unstable reduction, central intramedullary K-wiring from tip of DPX through IPJ for transfixation was done maintaining the congruency. The ideal position of IPJ for transfixation is neutral extension, but in this case in full extension, it was subluxing

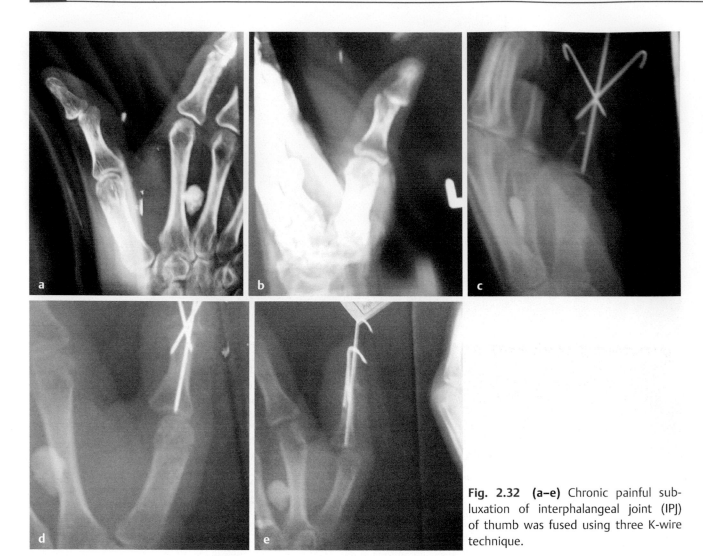

Fig. 2.32 (a–e) Chronic painful subluxation of interphalangeal joint (IPJ) of thumb was fused using three K-wire technique.

and on 30-degree flexion it was stable and congruent. In case of transfixation in this position one cannot get entry in to the medullary canal of PPX and fixation on the head of PPX is sufficient as shown in **Fig. 2.33a–h**. Here the K-wire was kept not more than 3 weeks because of worry of stiffness in flexion and early mobilization was started.

Case Scenario 2

Unreduced interphalangeal joint dislocation thumb. A 2-week-old neglected interphalangeal joint dorsal dislocation of the thumb was reduced by closed means with traction and manipulation. As the joint was unstable, it was secured by a joint transfixing intramedullary K-wire from the tip of DPX to PPX (**Fig. 2.34 a–e**).

Case Scenario 3

Dorsal fracture dislocation of DIPJ middle finger (**Fig. 2.35 a–h**). Small volar avulsion fragment (20% of articular surface) with dorsal dislocation of DIPJ. Here the dislocation was reduced but was found unstable; maybe it remained dislocated for a week's time. Hence after closed reduction and single intramedullary DIPJ transfixation, K-wiring was done for congruent reduction maintenance. The wire was removed at the end of 3 weeks, and 6 weeks postoperatively showed almost full recovery of movements.

Comminuted Distal and Proximal Phalanx Fracture Thumb (Fig. 2.36a–c)

Crush injury of the thumb resulted in the burst fracture of the DPX associated with splay out of fragments

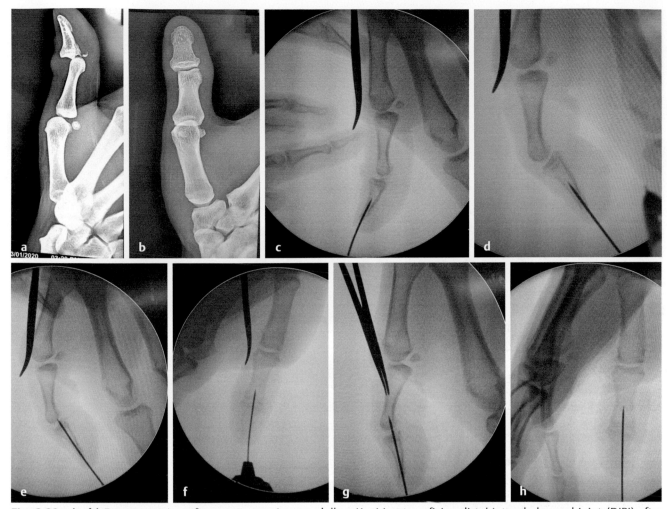

Fig. 2.33 (a–h) Demonstration of percutaneous intramedullary K-wiring transfixing distal interphalangeal joint (DIPJ) after closed reduction.

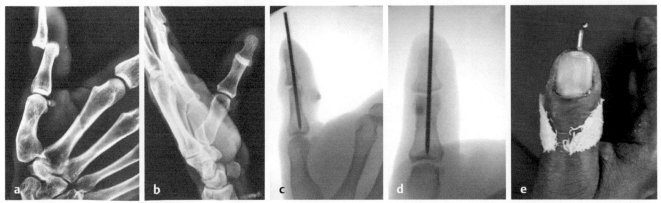

Fig. 2.34 (a–e) Interphalangeal joint (IPJ) dislocation stabilized in anatomical position with intramedullary K-wire.

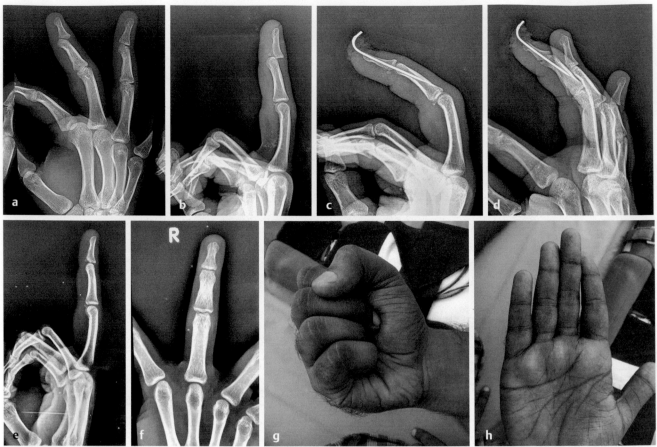

Fig. 2.35 **(a–h)** Dorsal fracture dislocation distal interphalangeal joint (DIPJ) reduced and fixed with simple intramedullary transfixation K-wire and its functional outcome.

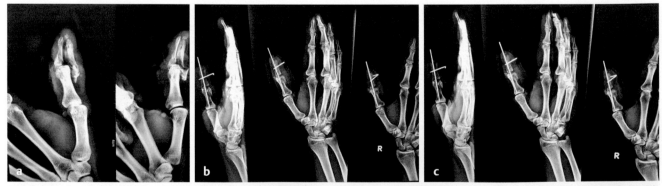

Fig. 2.36 **(a–c)** Comminuted burst fracture with shortening of distal phalanx (DPX) and proximal phalanx (PPX) of thumb reduced and restored the length by ligamentotaxis intramedullary K-wire and fragment-specific fixation.

in the sagittal plane. Here thin K-wire was used to pass from the tip of DPX intramedullary and passed through PPX and parked at the base using ligamentotaxis principle. This maintained the length and alignment. The split fracture was reduced by direct compression and fixed with a transverse 0.8-mm K-wire. This minimally invasive fixation without soft tissue damage

was important to save the thumb with precarious blood supply.

Fracture Dislocation of Distal Interphalangeal Joint Middle Finger (Fig. 2.37a–h)

An X-ray of a crush injury with a small burst wound dorsally revealed a unicondylar fracture head of MPX with

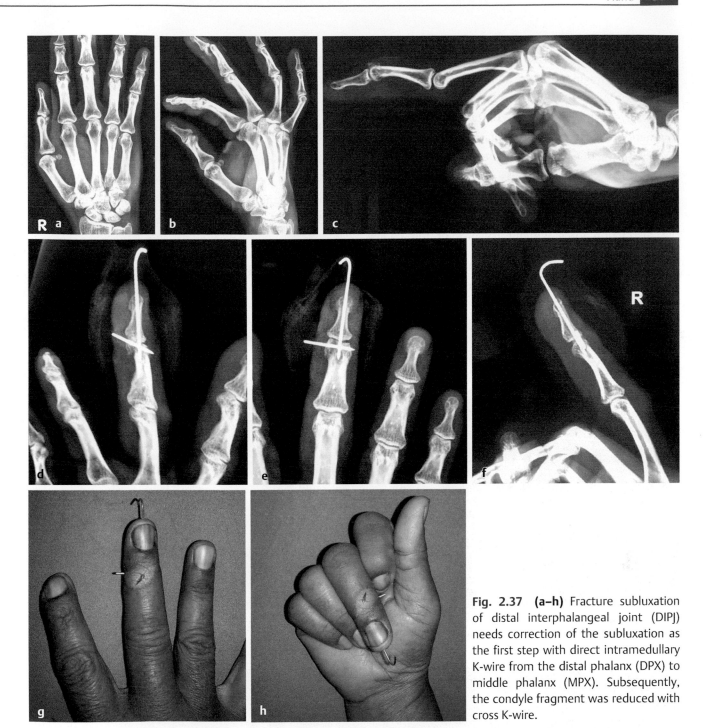

Fig. 2.37 (a–h) Fracture subluxation of distal interphalangeal joint (DIPJ) needs correction of the subluxation as the first step with direct intramedullary K-wire from the distal phalanx (DPX) to middle phalanx (MPX). Subsequently, the condyle fragment was reduced with cross K-wire.

DIPJ subluxation. This was reduced by a closed method but was found unstable due to the fracture. The unicondylar fracture of the head of MPX was reduced anatomically and fixed with a transverse 0.8-mm K-wire in slight flexion of DIPJ in order to enter in the safe corridor plane. Once this was anatomically reduced, mallet finger deformity persisted; hence a longitudinal intramedullary

K-wire was passed from the DPX tip to MPX in extension of DIPJ.

Comminuted Head of Middle Phalanx Fracture-Subluxation

Head of MPX fracture with split intra-articular fracture and subluxation was reduced by closed means and maintained by intramedullary K-wire passing from the tip of the DPX. In this case, the reduction and maintenance of the fragment in position was achieved by ligamentotaxis. As soon as the K-wire exits the DPX, traction of the finger with side-to-side compression will aid the fragments to fall in place. Maintaining the distraction force with traction, the wire was entered into the MPX medullary canal. The wire was parked at subchondral level of the base of the MPX by progressing slowly while drilling. Parking at subchondral hard bone maintains the distraction force without collapse or telescoping (**Fig. 2.38 a–e**).

Intra-Articular Fracture DIPJ Index Finger (Fig. 2.39a, b)

The fracture base of DPX and head of MPX were present. The fragments were reduced and stabilized with central single intramedullary K-wire using the principle of ligamentotaxis. The tip of the K-wire was parked at the MPX base in distraction mode.

Comminuted Intra-Articular Fracture DPX Base and Head of MPX (Fig. 2.40a, b)

Using the ligamentotaxis principle single snug fitting intramedullary K-wire from the tip of DPX spanning across DIPJ and parking in the base of MPX in distraction mode got the alignment and reduction of this fracture.

Fracture Subluxation of Interphalangeal Joint of Thumb (Partial Intra-Articular Fracture—Direct Fixation) (Fig. 2.41 a–e).

Unicondylar fracture of the MPX head can result in lateral deviation with subluxation of the joint. This needs anatomical reduction and it can be achieved by closed

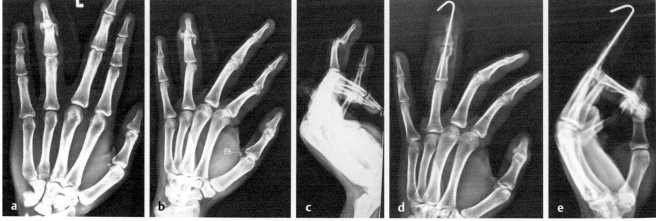

Fig. 2.38 (a–e) Comminuted head of middle phalanx (MPX) fracture with dislocation was reduced with intramedullary K-wire using ligamentotaxis principle by parking the tip of the wire in the subchondral bone of the MPX in distraction mode.

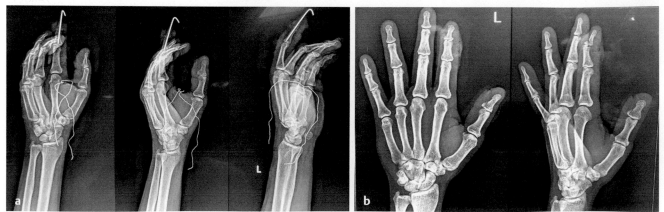

Fig. 2.39 (a, b) Fracture subluxation distal interphalangeal joint (DIPJ) index finger reduced and fixed with ligamentotaxis K-wire.

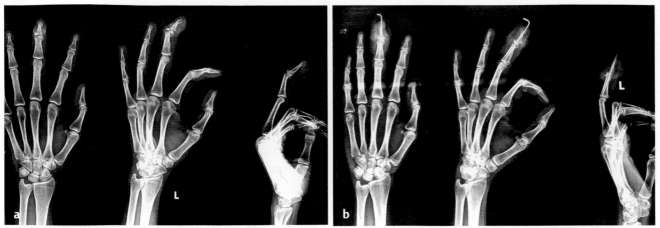

Fig. 2.40 (a, b) Multifragmented intra-articular comminution of distal interphalangeal joint (DIPJ) reduced and fixed with distraction K-wiring.

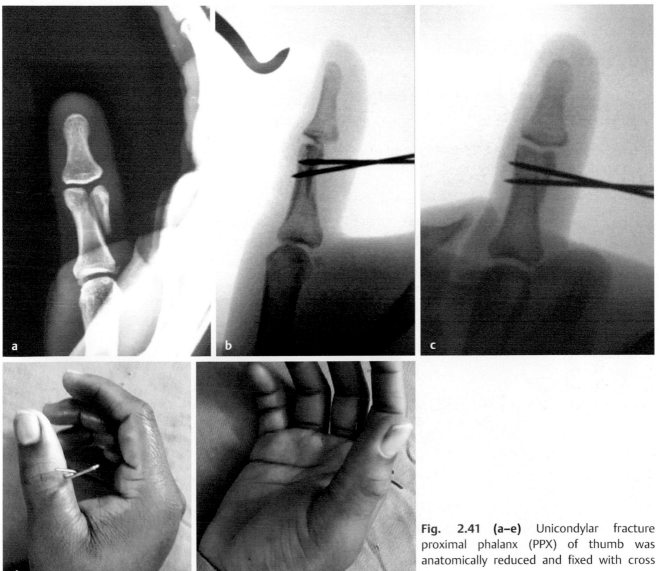

Fig. 2.41 (a–e) Unicondylar fracture proximal phalanx (PPX) of thumb was anatomically reduced and fixed with cross K-wires.

means by traction and pointed reduction clamp application with right orientation, (i.e., perpendicular to the fracture). Once anatomically reduced, this fracture was fixed with two ipsilateral entry divergent K-wires. K-wires were placed in divergent fashion as the fragment was big enough and in order to maintain rotational stability. Check for gentle active movement of thumb to assess stability.

Middle Phalanx

Unicondylar fracture head of MPX are treated by two methods:

1. Direct fixation of the fragment through the safe portal. This may be necessary in a grossly displaced fracture or rotary avulsed fragment where open reduction may be necessary, and in failed closed reduction methods.
2. Indirect fixation method where single thin intramedullary joint transfixation K-wire is used to correct the sagittal and coronal plane tilts.

Medial Condyle Head of Middle Phalanx of Ring Finger (Fig. 2.42a, b)

Here the fracture was reduced indirectly by transfixing the DIPJ in straight alignment with direct intramedullary K-wire from DPX tip to the base of MPX. Here a 1-mm intramedullary K-wire was used as thick wire

could splay the fracture fragment. Again ligamentotaxis principle of using thick K-wire is not necessary as only angular deformity needs correction. There is no necessity for thick wire as axial collapse or distraction is not a concern.

Lateral Condyle of Head of Middle Phalanx Fracture (Fig. 2.43a–h)

This is a displaced unicondylar fracture of head of MPX of middle finger. The radial aspect of the condyle was fractured with palmar tilt and displacement. This was reduced and fixed with single intramedullary joint transfixation K-wire as shown in **Fig. 2.43**. Here again thin K-wire was used to maintain the alignment and reduction.

Unicondylar Fracture Head of Middle Phalanx without Mallet Finger Deformity (Partial Intra-Articular Fracture—Direct Fixation)

The unicondylar fracture head results in angular deformity of the finger. One needs to analyze the personality of fracture for the placement of K-wire in safe zone of the head. On slight flexion the safe corridor gets wider. A small hypodermic needle is used to hold and manipulate the fragment for its reduction and to assess the direction of placement of K-wire. A 0.8-mm K-wire is used to transfix the fragment in an oblique direction just to engage the opposite cortex (**Fig. 2.44a–c**).

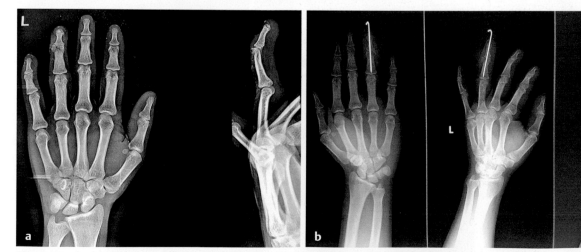

Fig. 2.42 **(a, b)** Indirect reduction of medial condyle head of middle phalanx (MPX) fracture with single intramedullary K-wire using ligamentotaxis principle.

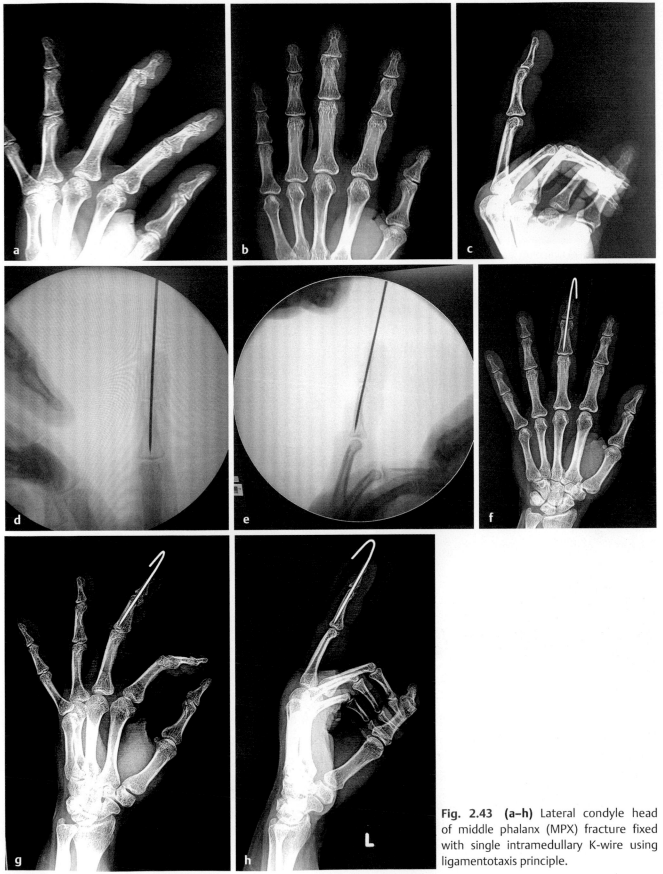

Fig. 2.43 (a–h) Lateral condyle head of middle phalanx (MPX) fracture fixed with single intramedullary K-wire using ligamentotaxis principle.

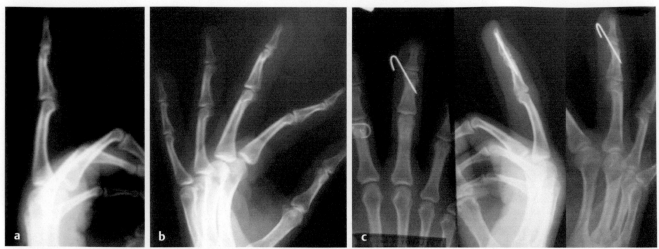

Fig. 2.44 (a–c) Unicondylar fracture with angular deformity was reduced and transfixed with cross K-wire through safe zone.

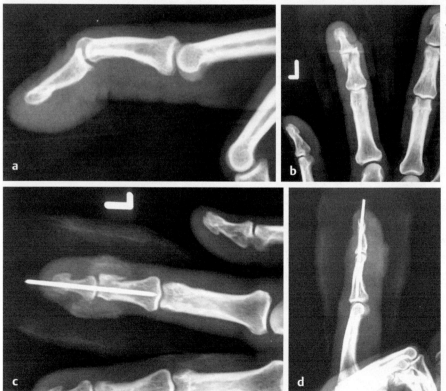

Fig. 2.45 (a–d) Fracture subluxation with mallet finger deformity was aligned and fixed with intramedullary K-wire.

Unicondylar Fracture Head of Middle Phalanx Fracture with Mallet Finger Deformity (Partial Intra-Articular Fracture—Indirect Fixation)

In this case, there is no dislocation or subluxation of the DIPJ, but mallet finger deformity is obvious. Hence, the mallet finger deformity was fixed with a straight intramedullary K-wire from DPX to MPX. As this did not displace the condylar head fragment, it got reduced as shown in **Fig. 2.45a–d** (this fixation was sufficient to address the fracture and the mallet finger deformity).

Unicondylar Fracture Middle Phalanx Head in a Child (Fig. 2.46a–c)

Medial unicondylar fracture of MPX head with subluxation of DIPJ in a child with angulation necessitated closed

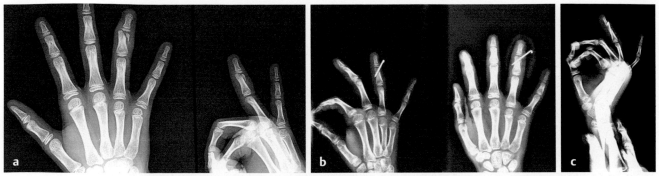

Fig. 2.46 (a–c) Unicondylar fracture head of middle phalanx (MPX) treated with direct K-wire fixation.

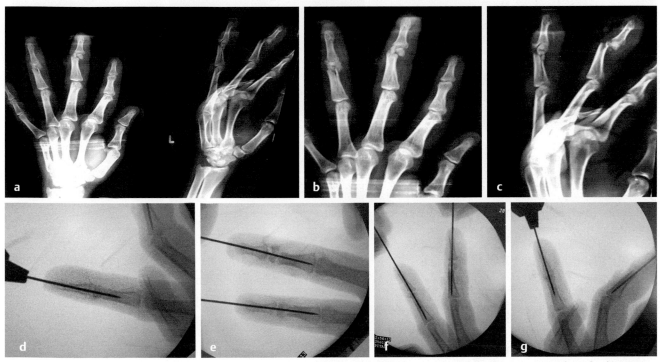

Fig. 2.47 (a–g) Comminuted fracture head of middle phalanx (MPX) ring and middle finger treated with distraction intramedullary K-wire.

reduction and K-wiring of the condyle through MPX safe corridor. This direct fixation achieved correction of the subluxation with articular congruity.

Comminuted Fracture Head of Middle Phalanx of Ring and Middle Finger (Fig. 2.47a–g)

Central intramedullary K-wire was passed from tip of DPX through DIPJ in to the comminuted head of MPX and parked in the base of MPX in distraction model using the ligamentotaxis principle. Similar procedure was done in ring finger.

Comminuted Head of Middle Phalanx Fracture in a Child (Fig. 2.48a, b)

Here intra-articular fracture of head and shaft of MPX was treated with single intramedullary snug fitting K-wire using the principle of ligamentotaxis from the tip of DPX across the DIPJ and parking in the subchondral bone at the base of MPX. Length, alignment, and fracture reduction were obtained.

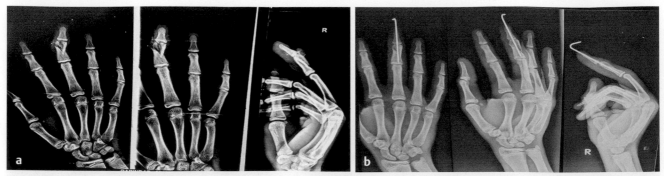

Fig. 2.48 **(a, b)** Comminuted head of middle phalanx (MPX) in a child treated with intramedullary distraction K-wiring.

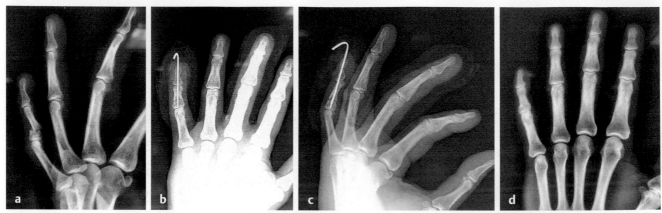

Fig. 2.49 **(a–d)** Single intramedullary K-wire for base of middle phalanx (MPX) fracture.

Middle Phalanx Shaft Base Fracture (Fig. 2.49a–d)

Displaced fracture base of MPX of little finger was reduced and fixed with intramedullary K-wire from the tip of the DPX through DIPJ and fracture site. After closed reduction of the fracture, the intramedullary wire was transfixed to the base of MPX. But if the fixation is inadequate, it can be transfixed on to the head of PPX in 0-degree extension of PIPJ.

Displaced Central Slip Avulsion Fracture (Partial Intra-Articular Fracture—Direct Fixation)

Large central slip avulsion fragment from the dorsal base of the MPX with minimal displacement can be repositioned on its bed by simple percutaneous reduction and direct K-wire transfixation as shown in **Fig. 2.50a, b**. A 0.8-mm K-wire can be passed through a small fragment manipulated using the wire as a joystick for perfect reduction in extension. The transfixing wire should not go beyond the opposite cortex as it may impale the flexor tendon. On-table examination, the active movement test is easy to rule out the proud K-wire on the volar aspect. A finger splint support in extension was given.

Central Slip Avulsion Fracture with Boutonniere Deformity (Partial Intra-Articular Fracture—Direct and Indirect Fixation)

The gross Boutonniere deformity is due to complete avulsion of central slip along with the collateral ligaments and capsule of the PIPJ. The joint is like a box (cube) with dorsal, radial, and ulnar capsule torn, resulting in obvious deformity. The joint transfixation K-wire in extension of the PIPJ was the most important K-wire to maintain congruent reduction and soft tissue healing. Additional K-wire to transfix the avulsed fragment was added as the fragment was big enough. In this case, the K-wire transfixing the joint was maintained for 5 weeks. Adjacent joint movements (DIPJ and MCPJ) were started in the immediate postoperative period (**Fig. 2.51a–c**).

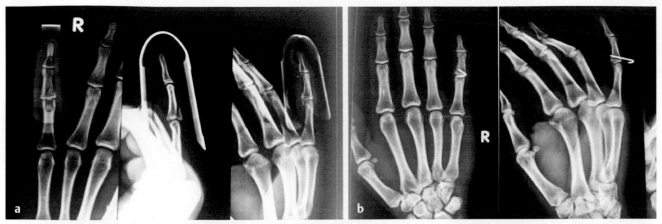

Fig. 2.50 (a, b) Central slip avulsion fracture fixed directly with K-wire.

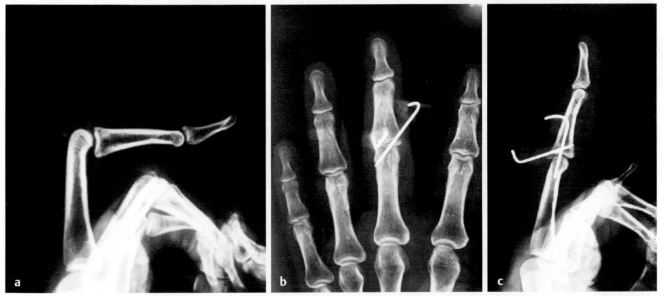

Fig. 2.51 (a–c) Central slip avulsion with Boutonniere deformity needed a joint transfixation K-wire in extension and direct transfixation of the avulsed fragment.

Fracture Medial Condyle Base of Middle Phalanx with Boutonniere Deformity (Direct Fragment Fixation) (Fig. 2.52a–f)

This fracture was reduced by closed means and direct transfixation of the medial fragment base of MPX was done with 1-mm K-wire. To prevent subluxation and Boutonniere deformity, joint transfixation single cross K-wire was done. This should be done from the intact lateral base of MPX to the head of PPX and maintained for a period of 6 weeks. The direct articular fragment fixation was removed at the end of 4 weeks.

Closed Central Slip Injury with Boutonniere Deformity (Fig. 2.53a–g).

Here a closed central slip injury was observed without avulsion fracture but with Boutonniere deformity. Maintaining the PIPJ in extension for 4 weeks for the healing of central slip with simultaneous active flexion of the DIPJ was important for normal excursion of extensor expansion. The functional position for immobilization of the PIPJ is 0-degree extension, when the collateral ligaments and volar plate are in their maximum stretched position. Eccentric attachment of the

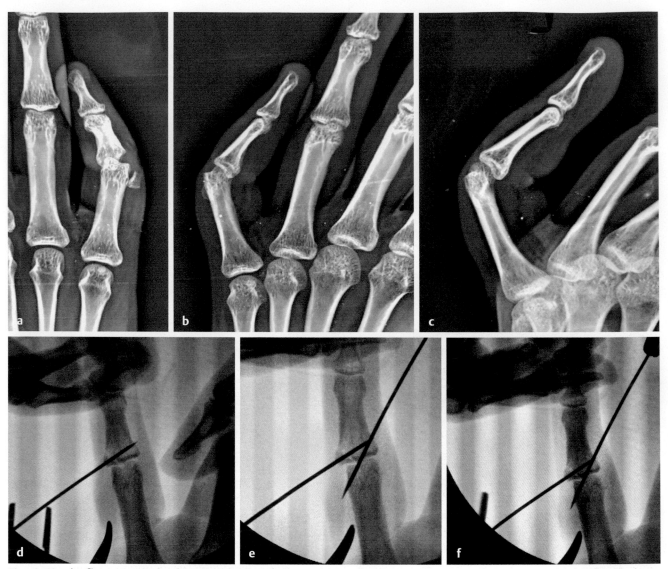

Fig. 2.52   (a–f) Intra-articular fracture middle phalanx (MPX) with Boutonniere deformity reduced and fixed with direct fragment specific K-wire and indirect joint transfixation K-wire for stability.

collateral ligaments on the PPX causes tightening in different range of motion. The button hole deformity is corrected and maintained in 0-degree extension by a transarticular cross K-wire in order to maintain the central slip in close contact and collateral ligaments in maximum stretched position.

Comminuted Fracture Base of Middle Phalanx with Volar Displacement (Fig. 2.54 a–g)

Severely comminuted intra-articular fracture base of the MPX showed the avulsion fragment of central slip with volar displacement, and it was reduced with traction

and direct external compression to align the fragment. A K-wire was passed from the DPX tip intramedullary into the DPX, DIPJ, MPX, PIPJ, and PPX head. The splaying out of the base was avoided by gentle compression of comminuted fragments while passing the wire with maximum traction. With ligamentotaxis principle, the fragments were maintained in distraction mode by carefully placing the K-wire in the subchondral area of the PPX (hard bone it cannot collapse or telescope) either distally or proximally in order to maintain the length of the finger. In this case, central slip avulsion fragment was only marginally displaced without needing a separate K-wire to transfix the fragment.

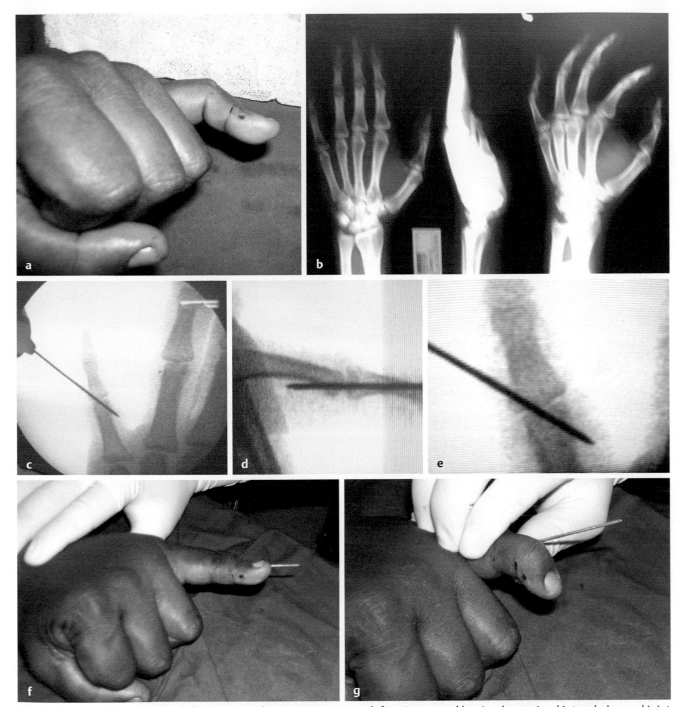

Fig. 2.53   (a–g) Closed central slip injury resulting in Boutonniere deformity treated by simple proximal interphalangeal joint (PIPJ) cross transfixation wire to aid in healing of the soft tissues and the active flexion of the distal interphalangeal joint (DIPJ) shown for excursion of extensor expansion without tethering. This movement brings the torn ligament together for good healing.

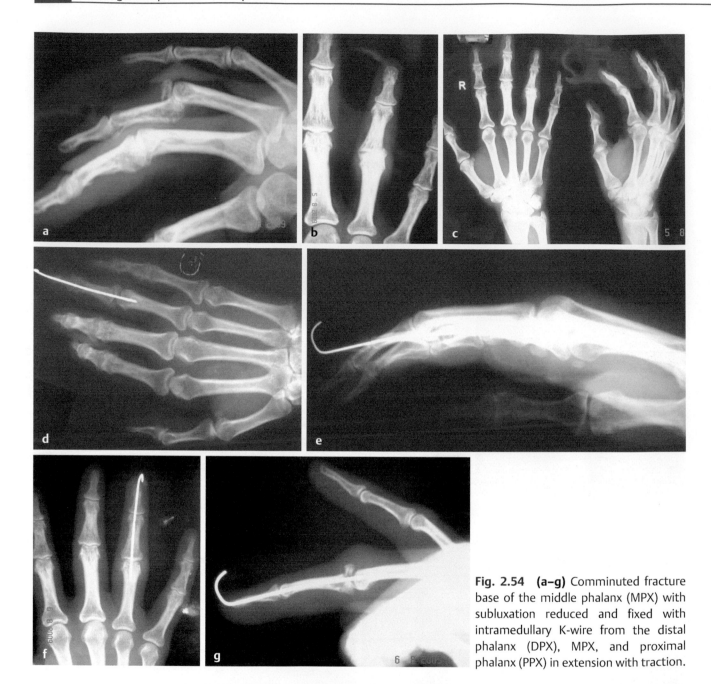

Fig. 2.54 (a–g) Comminuted fracture base of the middle phalanx (MPX) with subluxation reduced and fixed with intramedullary K-wire from the distal phalanx (DPX), MPX, and proximal phalanx (PPX) in extension with traction.

Volar Fracture Dislocation of PIPJ of Ring Finger (Fig. 2.55a–d)

Comminuted fracture base of MPX with dorsal avulsion fragment of central slip with volar subluxation of PIPJ with Boutonniere deformity was treated with single intramedullary K-wire from DPX using ligamentotaxis principle parking the tip at PPX head subchondral bone in distraction mode. Nice congruent reduction of the PIPJ was noted with falling back of all small comminuted

fragments. The K-wire was removed at the end of 4 weeks and active finger movements were started. Patient regained full movements at the end of 12 weeks.

Severely Comminuted Fracture Base of Middle Phalanx with Subluxation (Fig. 2.56 a–f)

Similar to the last case, intramedullary wire was passed from the DPX tip to MPX in a reduced position, and into the PPX to maintain the alignment. This K-wire was kept for a period of 4 weeks.

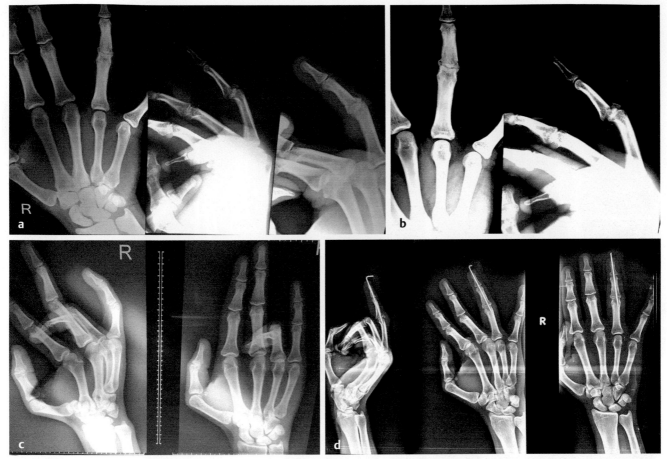

Fig. 2.55 **(a–d)** Volar fracture dislocation at proximal interphalangeal joint (PIPJ) reduced and fixed with distraction K-wiring technique.

Volar Proximal Interphalangeal Joint Dislocation with Central Slip Avulsion with Undisplaced Fracture Base of Proximal Phalanx Little Finger

After closed manipulation and reduction, the PIPJ was found unstable. Reduced PIPJ dislocation was maintained by an oblique K-wire passed from the MPX base, distal to proximal across the joint into the PPX head as shown in **Fig. 2.57a–f** keeping PIPJ in extension. Buddy strapping was given to treat the PPX base fracture. K-wire was left for 4 weeks, and DIPJ flexion and extension active movements were started from day 1 to prevent tethering of extensor expansion. The PIPJ was transfixed in extended position to keep the collateral ligaments at a maximum stretch so that further mobilization after K-wire removal becomes easy. At the end of 4 weeks, vigorous mobilization of PIPJ was started to prevent stiffness.

Volar Plate Avulsion Fracture Base of Middle Phalanx

PIPJ is the most commonly dislocated or subluxated joint among finger joints. The articular surfaces, collateral ligaments, extrinsic tendons, and volar plate act together to confer stability to this joint (**Fig. 2.58**). The volar plate, collateral ligaments, and central slip form a box around the PIPJ that imparts inherent strength. The PIPJ is the true epicenter of finger movement, whose position in the digital chain, between two long lever arms, makes it a particularly vulnerable joint.

The forces acting when such a fracture occurs is flexion at the PIPJ and extension at the DIPJ, causing the injury pattern known as the acute Boutonniere deformity (**Fig. 2.59**).

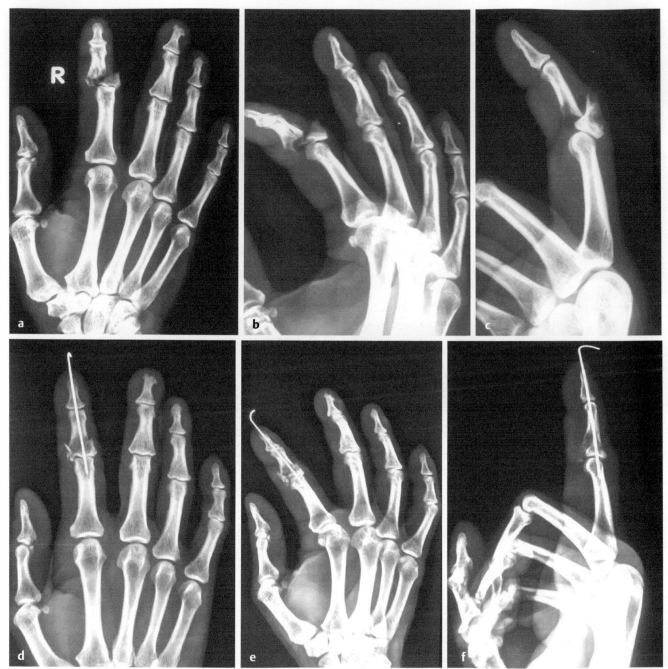

Fig. 2.56 **(a–f)** Fracture base of the middle phalanx (MPX) reduced and stabilized thoroughly with intramedullary K-wire from the distal phalanx (DPX), MPX, and proximal phalanx (PPX).

Dorsal Block K-Wiring

This technique has been effectively used for MPX volar plate avulsion fracture of PIPJ subluxation since late 1970s by Sugawa and colleagues in Japan, and N. J. Barton in Britain.

If closed reduction is possible under digital block, which is most often the case when presented within 2 weeks of injury, then closed reduction and dorsal block K-wiring can be done. If not, then open reduction and dorsal block K-wiring are done. Mobilization is started immediately after the procedure on table, to encourage the patient to continue further flexion from the extension block (**Fig. 2.60**).

It was noticed that it is not uncommon to have fractures with less than 25% joint surface involvement to

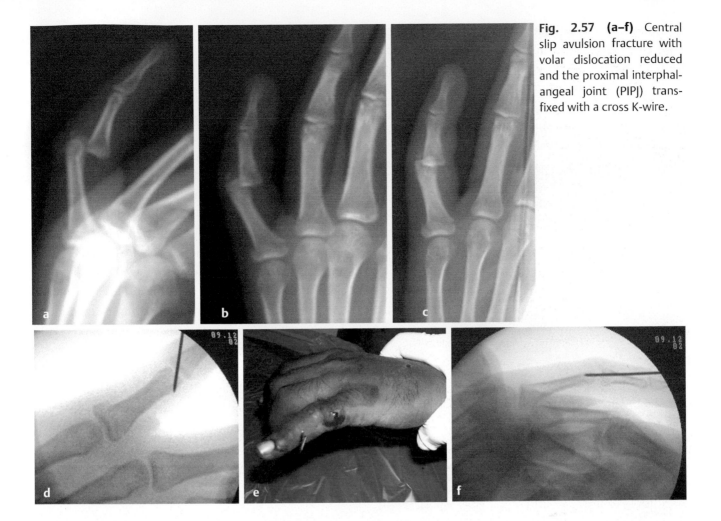

Fig. 2.57 (a–f) Central slip avulsion fracture with volar dislocation reduced and the proximal interphalangeal joint (PIPJ) transfixed with a cross K-wire.

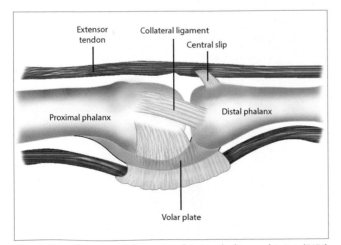

Fig. 2.58 Anatomy of proximal interphalangeal joint (PIPJ) and associated ligaments.

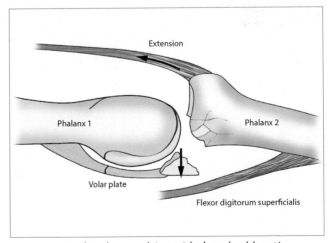

Fig. 2.59 Volar plate avulsion with dorsal subluxation.

lose reduction (dorsal subluxation) on course of conservative treatment, which might be because of extensive capsuloligamentous injury. Such cases were also treated by dorsal block K-wiring.

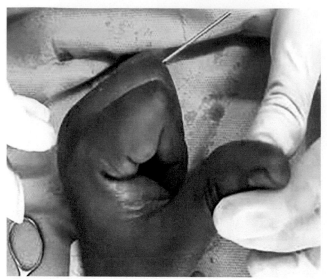

Fig. 2.60 Intraop demonstration of proximal interphalangeal joint (PIPJ) flexion of middle finger.

Operative Technique

All patients were treated under finger block. Constant traction was applied axially. Concentric reduction of PIPJ was achieved by flexion greater than 30 degrees; volar capsular avulsion fragment of the MPX base can be reduced by gentle manipulation. It is important to maintain PIPJ congruency by flexing the joint and it is not necessary to perfectly reduce the fracture.

During wire insertion, the DIPJ was flexed to relax the intrinsic mechanism, and the central slip tendon was pierced just proximal to its insertion with maximum flexion of both IP joints. Since the K-wire through central slip was pierced in the maximum flexed position, flexion of IPJ was possible in the postoperative rehabilitation phase with good excursion of extensor expansion. A dorsal blocking K-wire was introduced into the center of the PPX head along the long axis, preventing the dorsal movement and extension. The tip of the K-wire was then parked subchondrally. Congruent reduction was checked in lateral view under C-Arm guidance (**Fig. 2.61a–f** and **Video 2.1**).

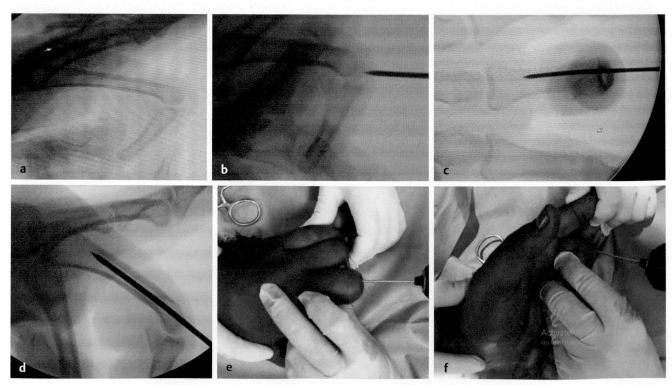

Fig. 2.61 **(a–f)** Closed reduction and dorsal blocking K-wire for indirect reduction of volar plate avulsion fracture.

Acceptance Criteria for Closed Reduction

- Rotational alignment along rest of fingers on further flexion.
- Concentric reduction of PIPJ on lateral view on fluoroscopy.

Further active flexion of PIPJ from the blocked extension position was checked on table. Normally full flexion is possible without any tethering or hindrance.

Weekly monitoring (clinical and radiological) with cleaning and dressing of pin site and hand physiotherapy was done.

Case Scenario 1

Volar plate avulsion fracture of the middle finger treated with dorsal blocking K-wiring and the follow-up of the patient with complete union and full range of movements (**Fig. 2.62a–l**).

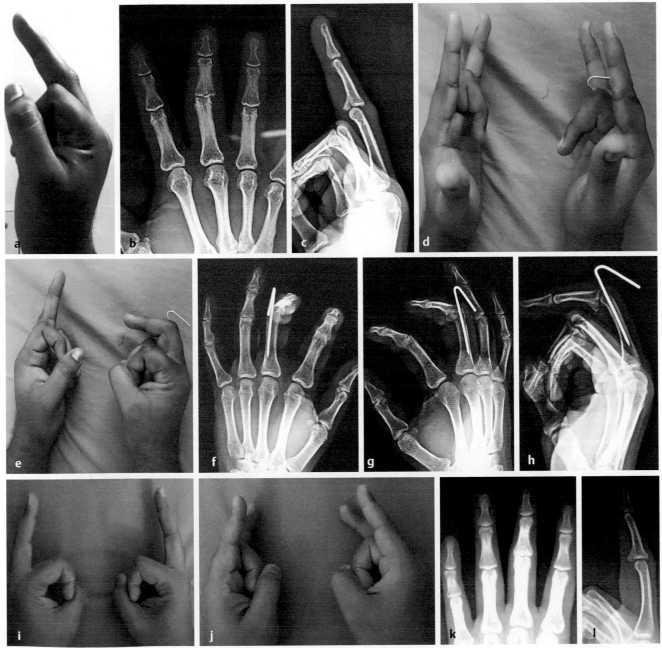

Fig. 2.62   (a–l) Preoperative and postoperative demonstration of dorsal blocking K-wire for volar plate avulsion fracture with functional outcome.

Case Scenario 2

Volar plate avulsion fracture of the ring finger treated with similar dorsal blocking K-wire technique and their follow-up (**Fig. 2.63a–r**).

Volar Plate Avulsion Fracture with Dorsal Dislocation of Proximal Interphalangeal Joint (Partial Intra-Articular Fracture—Indirect Fixation)

The volar capsular avulsion fragment of the MPX base can be reduced by maintaining 30- to 40-degree flexion of the PIPJ. However, when the intra-articular fracture fragment is associated with dorsal subluxation or dislocation of the PIPJ, the subluxation must be reduced to achieve good movements. A dorsal blocking K-wire was introduced into the center of the PPX head along the long axis, after reducing the dorsal subluxation of the PIPJ, preventing the dorsal movement and extension as shown in **Fig. 2.64a–c**. Congruent reduction was checked in lateral view. This is an indirect reduction technique for volar plate avulsion fragment. On-table examination showed that further flexion was full and easy, as shown in **Fig. 2.64d, e**, by performing a clenched fist.

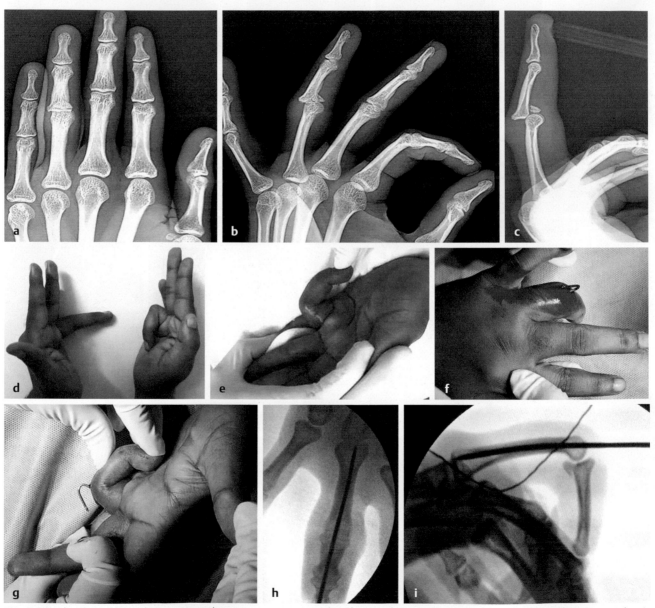

Fig. 2.63 **(a–i)** True lateral view is mandatory to appreciate volar plate avulsion with subluxation as other views may mislead. Technique of dorsal blocking K-wire demonstrated. *(Continued)*

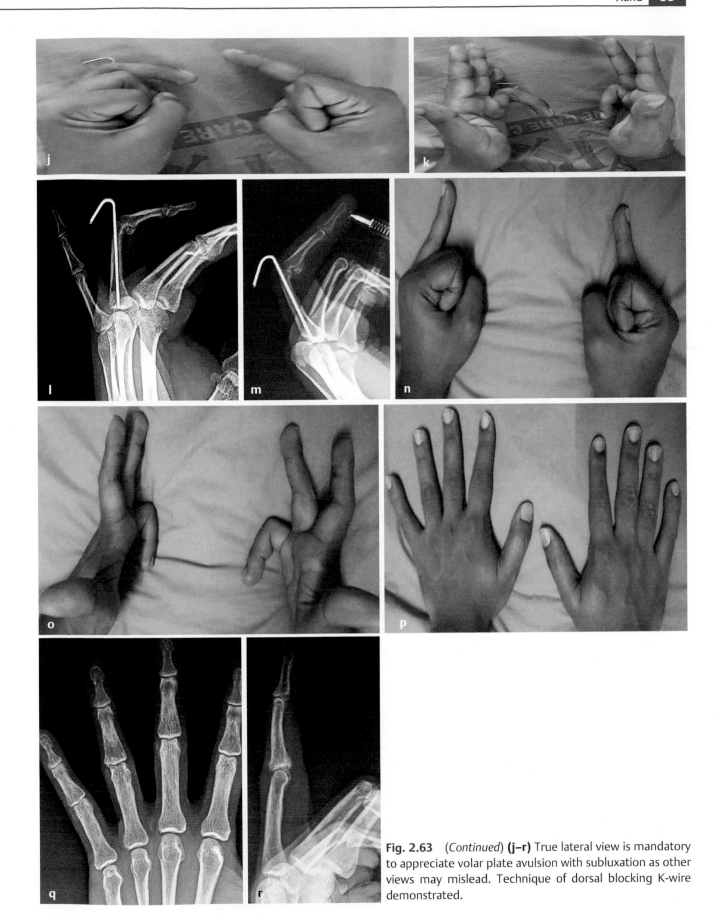

Fig. 2.63 (*Continued*) **(j–r)** True lateral view is mandatory to appreciate volar plate avulsion with subluxation as other views may mislead. Technique of dorsal blocking K-wire demonstrated.

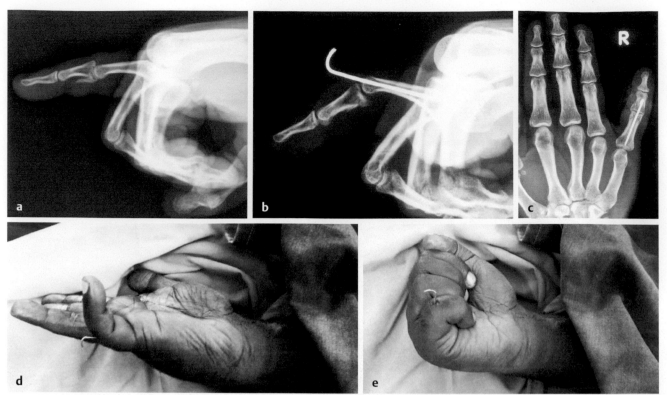

Fig. 2.64 (a–e) Volar plate avulsion fracture with dorsal subluxation reduced with dorsal blocking K-wire introduced through the proximal phalanx (PPX) head.

Extension was limited by the wire. After 3 weeks the K-wire was removed and gentle extension was started over a period of the next 3 weeks.

Fracture Neck of Middle Phalanx

Case Scenario 1

Middle phalanx neck fracture of middle finger (**Fig. 2.65a–d**). Fracture neck of MPX with angulation was corrected and fixed with single intramedullary K-wire from DPX tip through DIPJ. The hyperflexion at DIPJ was corrected by extending the DPX on head and passing the wire in neutral position (0-degree extension) of DIPJ and parallel to the dorsal cortex of MPX up to the fracture site. The fracture was reduced using the K-wire as a joystick and passed intramedullary to park at the base of the MPX.

Case Scenario 2

Displaced fracture neck of middle phalanx. The neck of MPX fracture can be manipulated and reduced by passing a K-wire from the DPX tip intramedullary.

Volar displacement of the MPX head is always difficult to reduce. It is easy to manipulate and reduce by performing joystick maneuver. The K-wire was passed from the DPX tip intramedullary and through the DIPJ. In this case, by flexing the DPX one can align the DIPJ in 0-degree extension in respect to the MPX head. This means that the wire enters the MPX head in the center and parallel to the longitudinal axis of the head in 0-degree extension. Once the wire entered the head in neutral position of DIPJ (0-degree extension), the head was manipulated to reduce over the proximal shaft fragment by traction in flexion in order to reach the fracture site and then did extension of the fragment for accurate reduction. Now the K-wire was advanced further intramedullary into the shaft of the MPX, checking under C-arm control in AP and lateral views (**Fig. 2.66a–f**).

Case Scenario 3

Neck of middle phalanx fracture in an adolescent boy. The boy had a cricket ball injury to his little finger that caused dorsally displaced fracture neck of the MPX. An intramedullary K-wire was passed from the DPX tip and

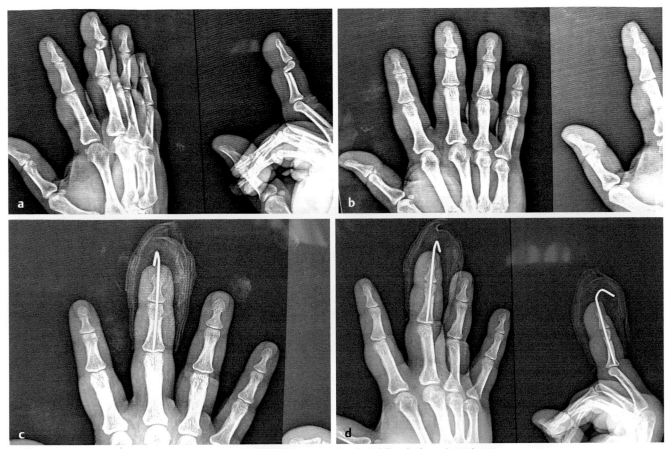

Fig. 2.65   (a–d) Intramedullary K-wire fixation for fracture neck of middle phalanx (MPX).

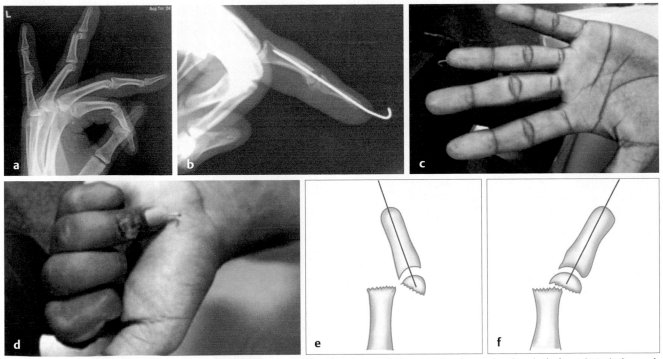

Fig. 2.66   (a–f) Middle phalanx (MPX) neck fracture fixed with intramedullary K-wire from the distal phalanx (DPX) through distal interphalangeal joint (DIPJ) and MPX fracture. **(c, d)** Technique of K-wire entry in to the head fragment of the MPX. **(e)** Hyperextension of DIPJ, **(f)** Normal extension DIPJ for entering with K-wire.

Vertical Split Fracture of Middle Phalanx

The die-punching machine injury caused burst longitudinal fracture of the middle and index finger with skin laceration. The fragments were splayed out with severe soft tissue contusion. The vertical split fracture of the MPX shaft was reduced by traction and circumferential compression with a pointed compression clamp or a pointed towel clip. The reduction was checked in C-arm scan and position was maintained with transverse 1-mm K-wire. This is just to transfix and should not shoot out more prominent off the far cortex. This type of unusual fracture pattern could not be fixed through a safe corridor entry. Additional parallel K-wires can be added if the fixation is inadequate (**Fig. 2.69a–g**).

Comminuted Fracture Shaft of Middle Phalanx

Case Scenario 1

Using the ligamentotaxis principle a snug fitting thick K-wire suiting isthmus of DPX was selected. Single intramedullary K-wire was passed from the tip of DPX, through DIPJ in to MPX and PIPJ maintaining the traction. The distraction mode was maintained by parking the tip of the wire on the hard subchondral bone of head of PPX. This maintains the reduction, length, and alignment. At the end of 4 weeks the wire was removed and flexion exercises for the finger was started. The final good functional result was shown at the end of 3 months both clinically and radiologically (**Fig. 2.70a–l**).

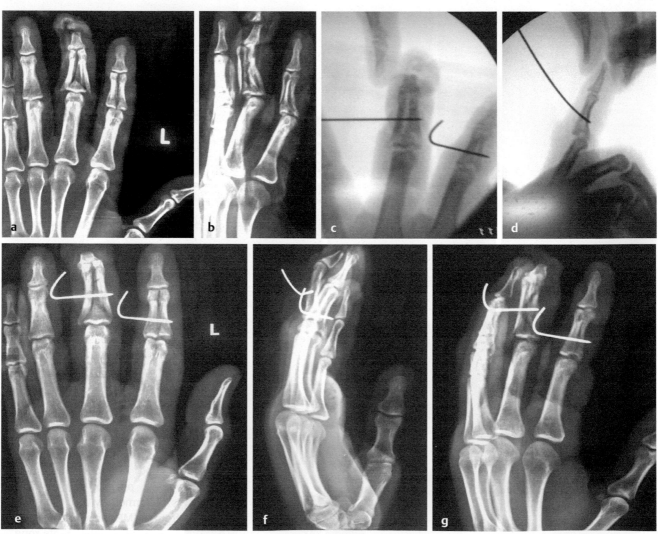

Fig. 2.69 (a–g) Vertical split fracture with splay out could be put together with one or two perpendicular K-wires.

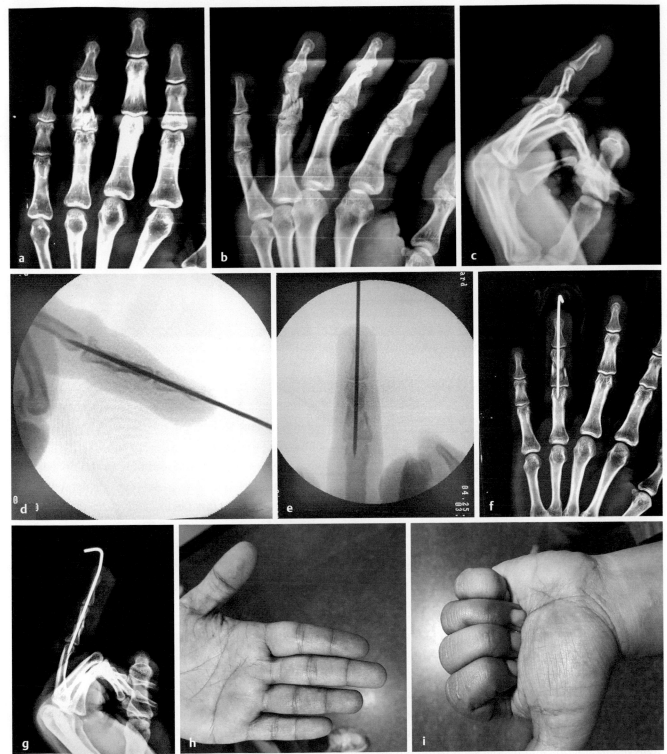

Fig. 2.70   (a–i) Intramedullary K-wire fixation using ligamentotaxis for comminuted fracture shaft of middle phalanx (MPX). *(Continued)*

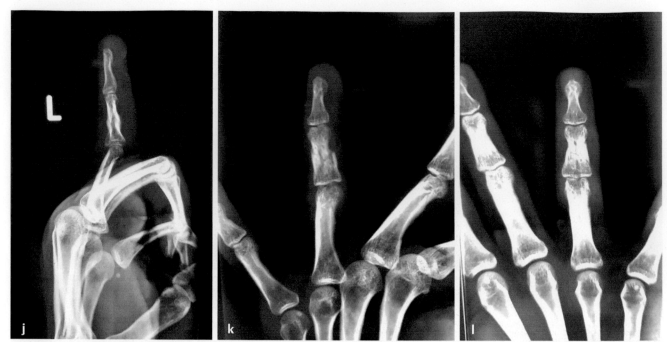

Fig. 2.70 (*Continued*) **(j–l)** Intramedullary K-wire fixation using ligamentotaxis for comminuted fracture shaft of middle phalanx (MPX).

Case Scenario 2

A central snug fitting intramedullary K-wire from the DPX tip to the subchondral base of PPX was done to get the length and alignment. The K-wire was removed at the end of 4 weeks and mobilization started. The fracture healed well with excellent functional outcome in spite of certain fragments being out of position at the end 6 months (**Fig. 2.71a–f**).

Displaced Partial Intra-Articular Fracture of Base of Middle Phalanx (Direct Fixation)

One should analyze the fracture pattern in three dimensions to know where the small intra-articular base fragment lies. In this case, the triangular base fragment is radial and volar in position. One wire was passed from dorsoulnar aspect of the MPX base into the small intra-articular volar radial fragment. The reduction was achieved by traction and by placing a pointed reduction clamp circumferentially around the finger at the level of the fracture gently, without causing damage to the volar digital vessels (it is not necessary to clip the pointed reduction clamp on the bone), and this would maintain the reduction. Another K-wire was passed from the volar radial fragment by keeping the finger in flexed position and aiming to dorsoulnar base. For the volar radial fragment, a K-wire was introduced only in the flexed position as this was important to prevent impalement of the soft tissue and to start flexion and extension of fingers from day 1 as shown in (**Fig. 2.72a–f**).

These wires should stop short as soon as it pierces the far cortex to prevent tethering. Patient should have pain-free early range of motion without any difficulty.

Middle Phalanx Base Comminuted Fracture with Joint Splay Out (Fig. 2.73a–c)

The displaced MPX base intra-articular fracture was treated with single intramedullary K-wire fixation using the ligamentotaxis principle. The preoperative and postoperative X-rays depict the anatomical reduction of these difficult fractures. The K-wire was removed at the end of 3 weeks and then mobilization of the small joints was encouraged. By the end of 6 weeks, good consolidation of the fracture and near normal movements of the finger were achieved.

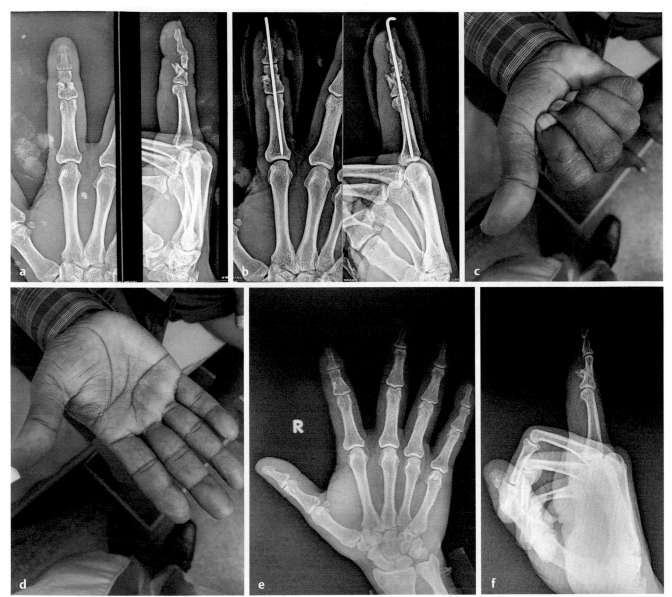

Fig. 2.71 **(a–f)** Ligamentotaxis K-wiring principle for comminuted middle phalanx (MPX) fracture with good functional outcome.

Displaced Middle Phalanx Base Fracture of Middle Finger

Displaced basal fracture shaft of the MPX was approached by K-wire passed from the DPX tip (safe corridor entry) intramedullary through the DIPJ and MPX. The fracture was anatomically reduced by traction and K-wire negotiated through the fracture assuming the central position in the medullary canal and parked engaging subchondrally at the MPX base for a snug fix (**Fig. 2.74a–e**).

Proximal Phalanx

Anatomical Consideration for Finger K-Wiring

The preferred entry point of single K-wiring of the PPX is from the ulnar side for the little and ring fingers and from the radial side for the index finger and thumb, respectively because of the orientation of extensor tendon. It can be done on either side for the middle finger. This is preferred to prevent impalement of extensor tendon on flexion and extension movement. Single K-wire has

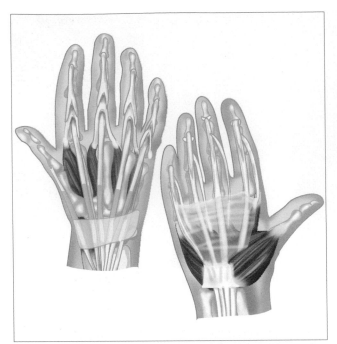

Fig. 2.75 Diagrammatic representation of the relationship of extensor tendon to the proximal phalanx (PPX) base.

corrects the rotation. A reduction thus achieved is classified as acceptable when there are less than 10 degrees of anteroposterior angulation, no mediolateral angulation, and no loss of height, collapse, or translation. A triangular wide area of safe zone for K-wire entry is present on the dorsolateral and dorsomedial aspect on either sides of the extensor tendon around the base of PPX, which gets wide open in flexion of MCPJ. This is the safe zone for entry of K-wire.

The isthmus level of shaft is the dependable determinant that aids in the selection of K-wire of an appropriate diameter. An ideal diameter of K-wire which is usually about 40% of the diameter is preferred for easy negotiation and snug fix. The commonly used sizes are 1-, 1.5-, 1.8-, or 2-mm-thick K-wires. Only the skin on either sides of the knuckle is incised with a No. 15 blade knife avoiding the sagittal band across the central extensor tendon. A mosquito forceps is employed for the soft tissue dissection. The PPX base is identified by lifting the PPX base as shown in **Fig. 2.76a, b**. This dorsal translation can be easily appreciated with practice and the PPX base becomes obvious for direct insertion of K-wire. Once the base of the PPX is reached, the first K-wire is passed from the dorsomedial or dorsolateral aspect directing intramedullary negotiating through the fracture into the

distal fragment but not completely to the final position (**Fig. 2.77a**). The second K-wire is then passed through the contralateral aspect of the base, intramedullary through the fracture site that ends up at the distal fragment. It is stopped short of the final position (**Fig. 2.77b**). With fluoroscopic guidance final adjustments are made to achieve the optimal reduction correcting angulation, thus helping the restoration of alignment and rotation. Both the K-wires are progressively driven to get engaged at the subchondral bone of the head of PPX. Care has to be taken in regard to the direction of the K-wires. A near parallel placement of the wires in more distal fractures such as those seen in the neck fracture is much needed to get proper engagement. There may also be some circumstances where crisscross placement too would not much hinder the functional outcome (**Fig. 2.77c, d**). This technique provides an adequate rotational stability, eliminating the need for entry into the opposite cortex. Because there is no piercing of the far cortex, there is no impalement of soft tissue by the tip of the K-wire. The practice of dual intramedullary K-wiring ensures a snug fit while allowing a greater degree of range of movements and better control over both the bending and rotational forces. It is prudent to ensure that whole range of active movement of the finger (on-table active flexion test) is preserved while simultaneously ruling out any soft tissue impalement and any other injury. Care must be taken to check for full flexion and for any rotational deformity. Although a skin release incision is not always indicated, it may be occasionally necessary in order to fend off any possibility of skin or soft tissue tethering. The K-wire is bent and cut. Sterile antiseptic dressing using povidone iodine is done.

Postoperative Care and Rehabilitation

The patients were encouraged to practice their full range of movements postoperatively. The exercise started intraoperatively while checking for range of movements will help in installing more confidence in patients to begin their rehabilitations as early as the first postoperative day. The rehabilitation was commenced and supervised by the hand physiotherapist. The patients were put on alternate day sessions and continued until a full fist could be made by the patients. In-hospital supervised physiotherapy once a week along with regular weekly

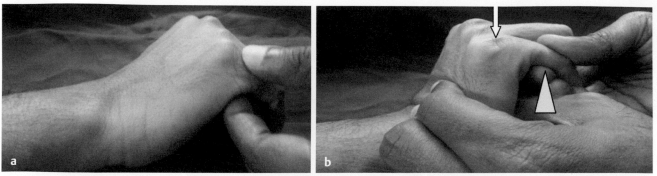

Fig. 2.76 (a, b) Demonstration of how to visually appreciate the proximal phalanx (PPX) base by lifting up as shown for easy insertion of K-wire through the base.

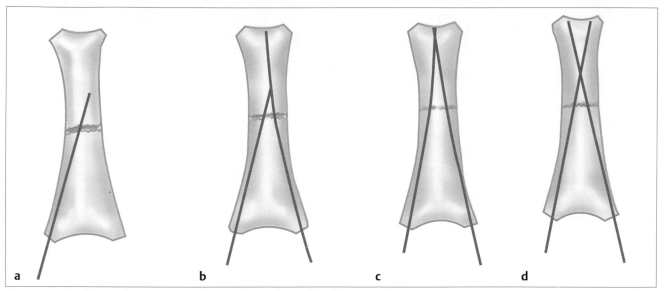

Fig. 2.77 (a–d) Line diagram representing the method of double K-wire insertion.

dressings was done for a period of 4 weeks. The K-wires were removed in OPD at the end of 4 weeks except in comminuted/open fractures where it was delayed for 4 to 5 weeks. Radiological evidence of healing was not taken into account for the removal of K-wire.

However, the radiographs were performed on regular intervals usually on the first postoperative day and then at 3, 6, 12, and 24 weeks to look for any loss of position, collapse, and radiological healing. Patients were allowed to start out delicate activities involving operated digits at the end of the third week. Rehabilitation was slowly stepped up until sixth postoperative week when the patients were encouraged to perform any activity to its full extent except load bearing (**Fig. 2.78a–i).**

If the swelling of the finger is too much, and if the fracture is too proximal in PPX it is easy to reduce with a gauze around the base of the finger to lift in the flexed position to reduce the fracture as shown in **Fig. 2.79.**

Case Scenario 1

Fracture midshaft PPX middle finger displaced treated by antegrade double intramedullary K-wire fixation (**Fig. 2.80a, b**).

Case Scenario 2

It is a case of malunited proximal phalanx fracture of ring finger.

A wrongly performed surgery for fracture PPX that led to malunion, resulting in stiff finger: it is unpardonable to do a procedure such as this that will ruin the hand function. This was removed, and adjacent joints were manipulated to ease up the stiffness (**Fig. 2.81a**).

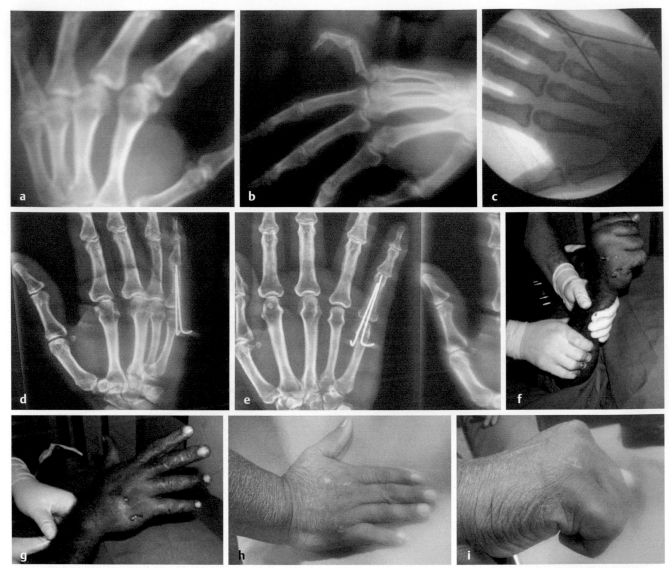

Fig. 2.78 **(a–e)** Displaced fracture proximal phalanx (PPX) of the little finger fixed with two intramedullary K-wires from the base. **(f, g)** On-table test showing full flexion and extension. Displaced fracture PPX of the little finger fixed with two intramedullary K-wires from the base. **(h, i)** A 4-week postoperative view shows almost full range of movements (a week after the removal of K-wire).

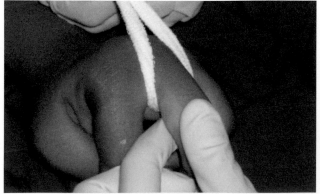

Fig. 2.79 The base of proximal phalanx (PPX) can be lifted up using a gauze for easy reduction and entry of K-wire.

Two cross K-wires were passed after an open anatomical reduction and internal fixation from the PPX base with double intramedullary K-wires (**Fig. 2.81b**).

Case Scenario 3

The principle of passing a K-wire from the base of PPX (safe corridor) was followed in multiple proximal phalanx fracture.

Fracture PPX of the Little and Ring Fingers with rotational deformity (**Fig. 2.82a–e**).

Here two K-wires on either side of the PPX base were passed to give rotational stability in ring finger.

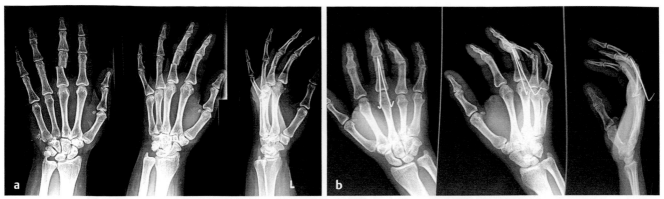

Fig. 2.80 **(a, b)** Antegrade double intramedullary K-wire fixation for proximal phalanx (PPX) transverse midshaft fracture.

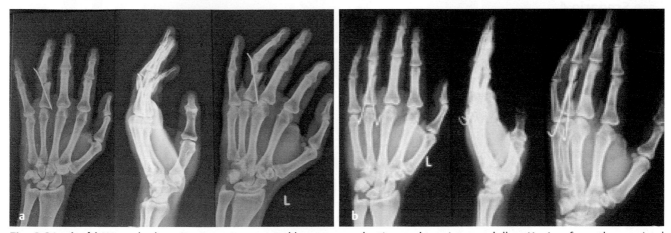

Fig. 2.81 **(a, b)** Wrongly done K-wire was corrected by proper reduction and two intramedullary K-wires from the proximal phalanx (PPX) base.

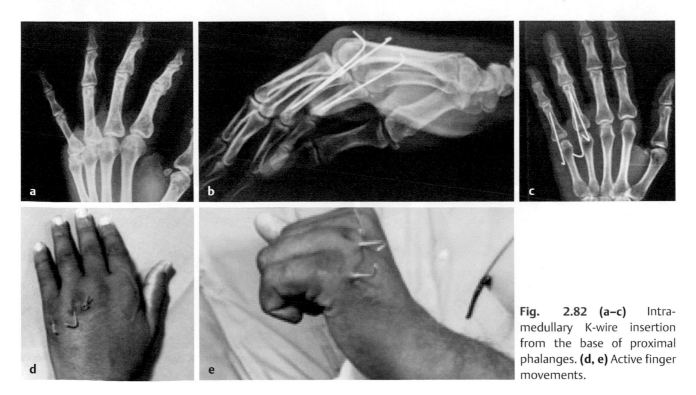

Fig. 2.82 (a–c) Intramedullary K-wire insertion from the base of proximal phalanges. **(d, e)** Active finger movements.

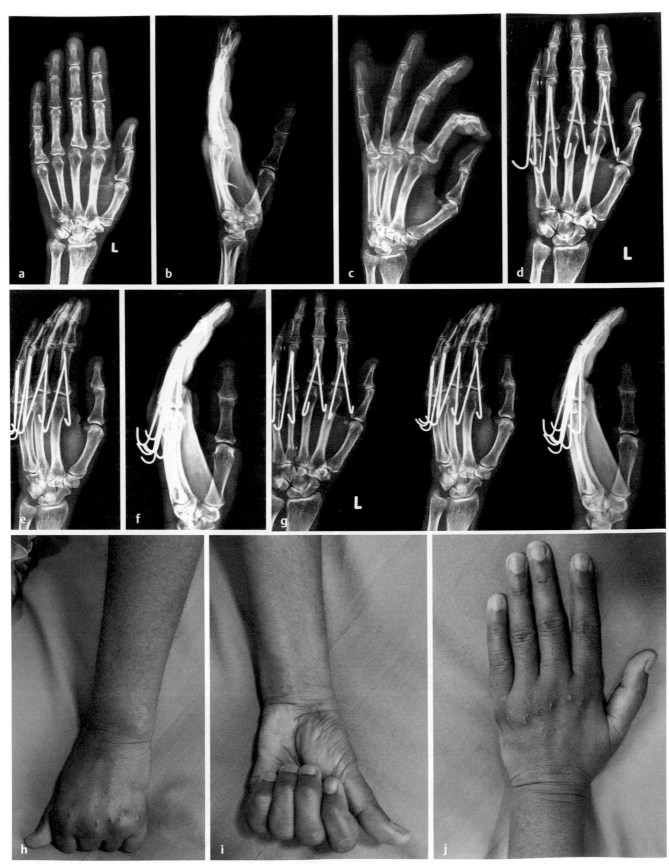

Fig. 2.85 **(a–j)** Multiple proximal phalanx fracture treated with antegrade double intramedullary K-wire.

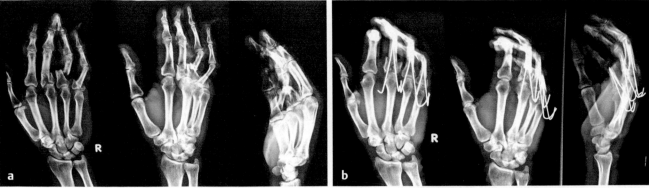

Fig. 2.86 (a, b) Intra-articular fracture base of proximal phalanx (PPX) F3 and F5 along with shaft PPX fracture of F4 treated with double intramedullary antegrade K-wiring.

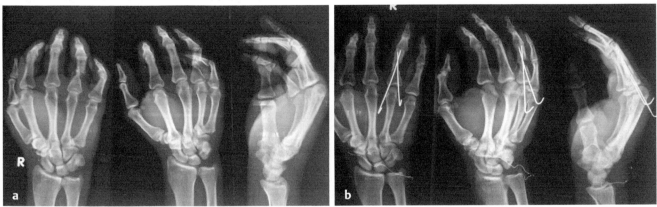

Fig. 2.87 (a, b) Two cross K-wires from the base are necessary to stabilize a transverse fracture proximal phalanx (PPX).

intramedullary in the distal fragment. We have found this technique is still worthy on these special situations as well.

Case Scenario 8

It is Open Comminuted Proximal Phalanx Fracture of Ring Finger

In **Fig. 2.87a**, the radiograph shows ring finger PPX fracture with severe comminution extending into the distal shaft and PPX head. Two crossed K-wires were passed from the PPX base, preferably more parallel on either side of extensor tendon (**Fig. 2.87b**).

Technical Tip

Convergent K-wires will fail to fix the distal fragment as wire exits at the fracture site, and one cannot cross the fracture site. K-wires passed parallel to the shaft can cross the fracture site comfortably to fix into the distal fragment (**Fig. 2.88**).

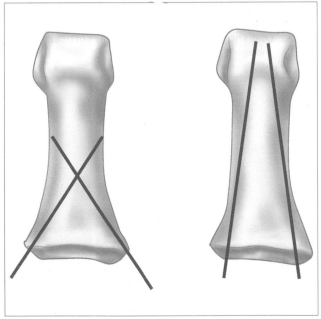

Fig. 2.88 Convergent K-wire entry from the base of the bone will abut the shaft not entering the distal part. Parallel K-wire will allow the tip to reach the distal part.

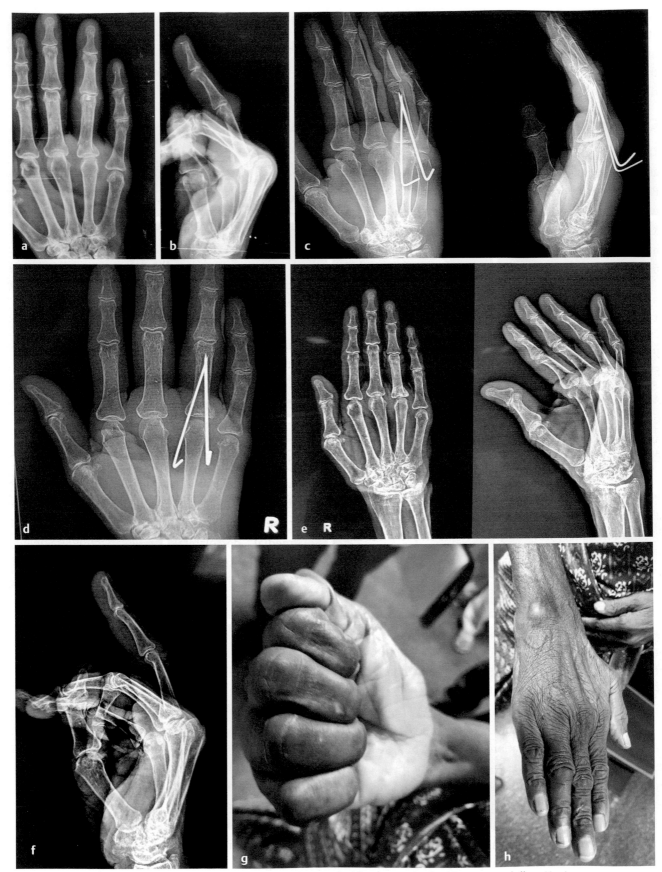

Fig. 2.94 **(a–h)** Fracture proximal phalanx (PPX) base treated with antegrade double intramedullary K-wire.

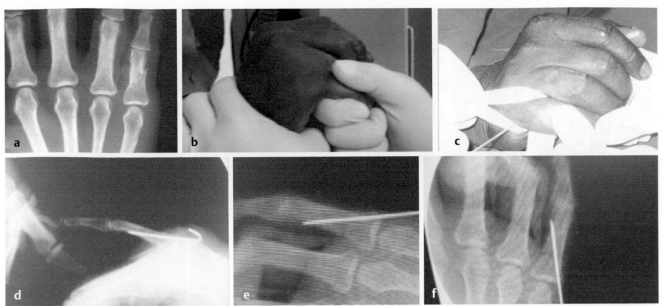

Fig. 2.95 **(a–f)** Reduction technique and insertion of K-wire from the base is demonstrated. If single K-wire is used, this wire should transfix the opposite cortex for rotational stability as shown.

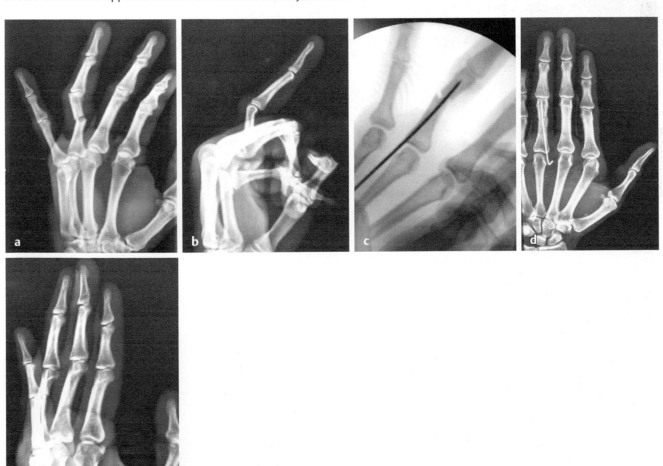

Fig. 2.96 **(a–e)** Single thick intramedullary K-wire can angulate the fracture as shown and was rectified by swapping with a thin K-wire or with two K-wires from the base in the conventional manner.

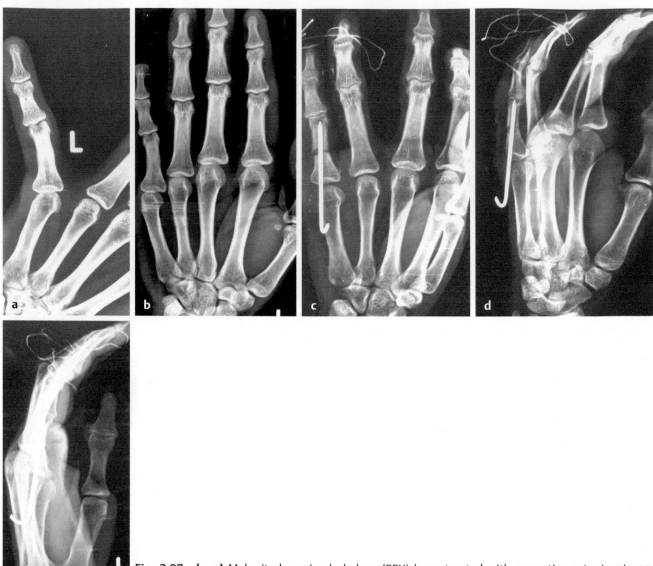

Fig. 2.97 (a–e) Malunited proximal phalanx (PPX) bone treated with corrective osteotomty and thick single intramedullary K-wire from the ulnar base to correct the alignment.

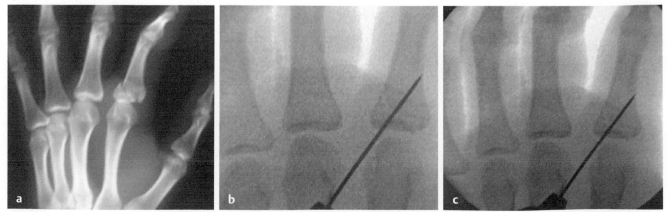

Fig. 2.98 (a–c) K-wire from the small fragment transfixing the distal large fragment proximal phalanx (PPX) correcting palmar subluxation.

Another less desirable alternative method is direct oblique K-wiring after perfect reduction. Here respecting the soft tissues, one should use the safe portal of entry with minimal soft tissue impalement as demonstrated by "on-table active finger flexion test." Sometimes this may not be possible in direct K-wiring and it is a suboptimal method of fixation.

At the Distal One-Third

Long oblique fracture in the middle and distal third junction of the PPX can be stabilized by maintaining its length by clamping the soft tissues gently around the fracture site with a towel clip after exerting longitudinal traction of the finger. Once it is anatomically reduced, the fracture is stabilized with two oblique K-wires passed perpendicular to the fracture, as shown in **Fig. 2.99a–c**. Active finger flexion and extension are tested to prevent tethering.

At the Middle One-Third

Long oblique fractures are intrinsically unstable and there is a tendency to slide down, shorten, and go for a rotational deformity. The fracture can be anatomically reduced by longitudinal traction with the PIPJ in flexion. A towel clip can be gently applied wrapping the finger from outside with gentle squeeze for maintaining reduction without compromising the finger circulation, and

transfixation with two K-wires is done. The fracture reduction was checked after releasing the clamp. Two parallel or divergent K-wires were passed from distal to proximal fragment perpendicular to the fracture line as shown in **Fig. 2.100a–e**.

These wires were passed in midlateral position poking the soft tissues in full extension of the PIPJ so that in postoperative period, full flexion at the PIPJ will be easy. The K-wire should not be left prominent at exit as this can impale the flexor or extensor tendon. One should use at least two K-wires to prevent rotation. Always check for active full flexion and extension of the fingers by active movements performed by the patient as shown in **Fig. 2.101a, b**. A 9-month postoperative view shows full range of movements clinically and radiologically with healed fracture (**Fig. 2.102a–c**).

Long Spiral Fracture Neck of Proximal Phalanx

Displaced long spiral fracture with shortening at the neck of PPX fracture leads to tethering of the collateral ligaments and restriction of flexion. This needs anatomical reduction and stabilization. Reduction can be accomplished by a longitudinal traction with circumferential pointed reduction clamp to squeeze gently for a perfect reduction as shown in the previous example. The safe zone of entry for transfixation wire for this type of fracture is through the PPX head as shown in **Fig. 2.103a, b**, so that immediate flexion and extension can be started.

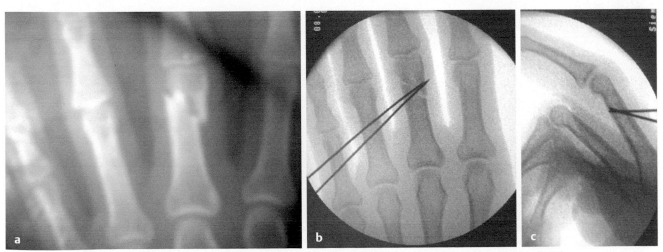

Fig. 2.99 **(a–c)** Two side-to-side K-wires used to transfix the short oblique fracture proximal phalanx (PPX).

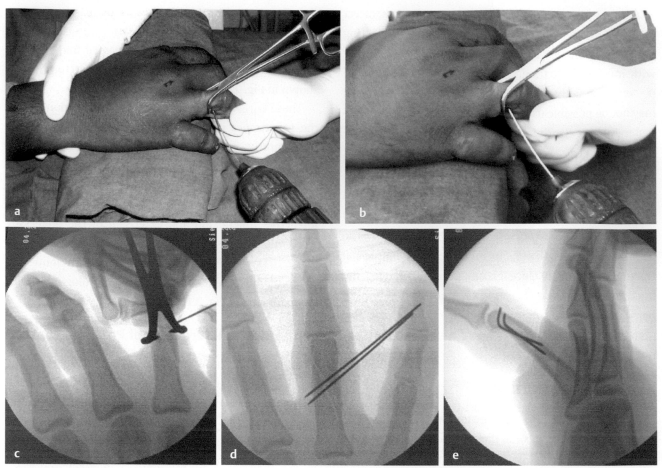

Fig. 2.100 **(a–e)** Pointed reduction clamp applied circumferentially to reduce the long spiral fracture, and two side-to-side direct transfixation K-wires were passed.

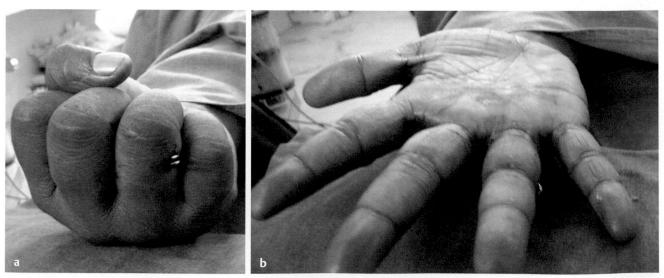

Fig. 2.101 **(a, b)** Checking for the range of movements after K-wire transfixation.

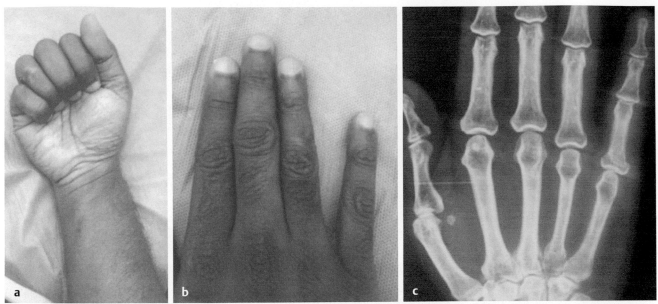

Fig. 2.102 **(a–c)** A 9-month postoperative healed fracture showing full flexion and extension clinically.

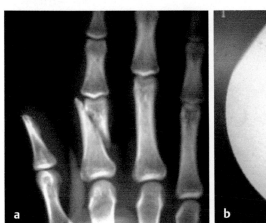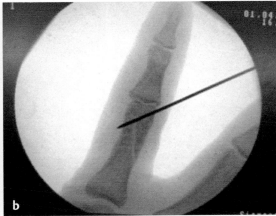

Fig. 2.103 **(a, b)** Long spiral fracture reduced and transfixed with a K-wire from the head pointing perpendicular to the fracture.

Long Oblique Fracture Shaft of Proximal Phalanx Ring Finger (Fig. 2.104a–k)

The long oblique fracture shaft of PPX ring finger with angulation and rotational deformity was corrected by traction and flexion of adjacent fingers together at MCPJ for proper rotational alignment. This fracture can be treated by either direct fixation through head of PPX after anatomical reduction with pointed clamp or by antegrade double intramedullary K-wire fixation. Here the second method was adopted as anatomical reduction was not possible by closed method. Double intramedullary almost parallel K-wires were inserted from the base of PPX parking subchondrally after proper reduction and rotational alignment control as described above. Mild translation was accepted. The wire was removed at the end of 3 weeks, and follow-up 2 months postsurgery demonstrates excellent function with good radiological healing.

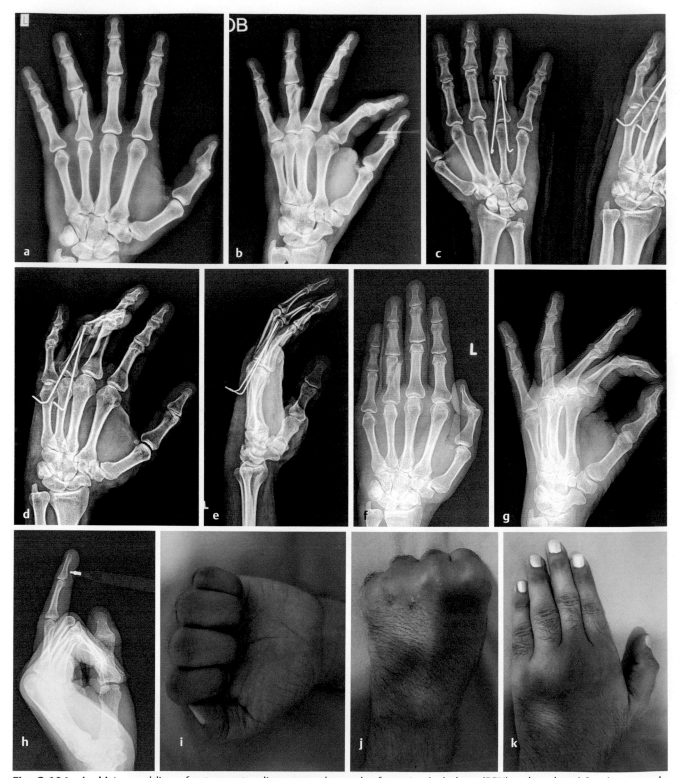

Fig. 2.104 **(a–k)** Long oblique fracture extending up to the neck of proximal phalanx (PPX) reduced and fixed antegrade double intramedullary K-wire with parking at PPX head.

Severely Comminuted Proximal Phalanx Base Intra-Articular Fracture Ring Finger (Fig. 2.105a–i)

Following the ligamentotaxis principle, the intramedullary K-wire entered from the tip of PPX was parked on the metacarpal at 70-degree flexion of MCPJ transfixing the joint in the distraction mode. It is preferable to start from the tip of the finger DPX with IPJ in extension but wrong direction may not allow threading of all phalanges before passing through MCPJ as it happened here. Hence K-wire entered from PPX head intramedullary and parked in metacarpal in distraction mode at 70-degree flexion. Good alignment and reduction were obtained.

Displaced Comminuted Fracture Base of Proximal Phalanx Index Finger

Comminuted fracture base of PPX resulted in gross displacement with subluxation. Traction brought these fragments into reasonable alignment. As shown in **Fig. 2.106a–i**, the K-wire was passed from the second metacarpal head pointing toward the center of medullary canal in 70-degree flexion. One should avoid impaling the extensor tendon by manually pushing the tendon aside of the entry point. Maintaining the distraction and reduction of the fragment by the ligamentotaxis principle, the second MCPJ was transfixed at 70-degree angle and intramedullary positioning of K-wire into the PPX was done to the subchondral bone of the PPX head. This parking position is crucial to prevent collapse of the PPX and again the wire should not pierce the head as the distraction tension will be lost. Good reduction was achieved by this technique and wire was removed at the end of 4 weeks period and started on MCPJ movements.

Thumb Fracture

Unicondylar Fracture Radial Aspect of Head of Proximal Phalanx Thumb (Partial Intra-Articular Direct Fixation)

Displaced unicondylar fracture head of the PPX needs anatomical reduction to prevent deformity and angulation. K-wire was engaged first over the fractured condyle. The articular step was reduced and transfixed to the opposite condyle using the K-wire as a joystick.

If the fixation was inadequate, one more K-wire could be added depending on the size of the fragment and preferably in a divergent fashion (**Fig. 2.107a–c**).

Unicondylar Fracture Ulnar Aspect of Head of Proximal Phalanx of Thumb (Partial Intra-Articular Direct Fixation)

A 20-day-old ulnar condyle of PPX head fracture, which was maluniting, was reduced by open reduction through midlateral approach from the ulnar side. The rotated fragment was reduced anatomically and under direct vision two K-wires were passed from the head to the shaft transversely and obliquely in a divergent fashion through the safe corridor. Range of movements was checked and skin was closed with interrupted 3-0 Ethilon (Ethicon, Inc., Somerville, New Jersey) (**Fig. 2.108a–f**).

Ulnar Collateral Avulsion Fracture of Proximal Phalanx Base of Thumb

Acute injury to ulnar collateral ligament of the thumb is well known in skiing sports or fall on outstretched hand known as Stener lesion. However, avulsion fracture is not uncommon, and if the fragment is big enough, it can be reduced by open method and internal fixation done with a K-wire (**Fig. 2.109a–e**).

Radial Collateral Ligament Avulsion Fracture of MCPJ Thumb (Fig. 2.110a–e)

Displaced lateral collateral avulsion fragment from PPX thumb base of MCPJ was reduced using a 18-gauge hypodermic needle. Once reduced 1.2-mm K-wire was used to transfix the fragment on to the bed and secured to the opposite cortex as depicted in **Fig. 2.110**. A thumb splint was given for a period of 4 weeks.

Open Unicondylar Fracture Head of Proximal Phalanx Thumb

Direct injury to the thumb can result in an open unicondylar fracture subluxation of the PPX head. The osteochondral small fragment was avascular with little soft tissue attachment. Replacing this fragment may cause infection and avascular necrosis. This loose fragment was excised and joint stabilized with intramedullary K-wire

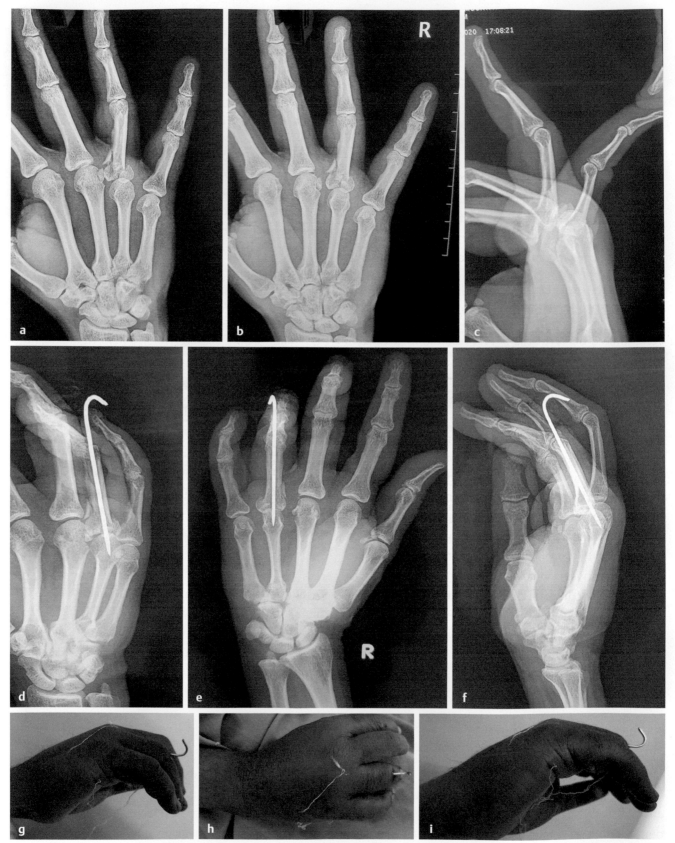

Fig. 2.105 **(a–i)** Intra-articular fracture of the proximal phalanx (PPX) base treated by ligamentotaxis principle with K-wire from PPX head intramedullary parking on the head of metacarpal.

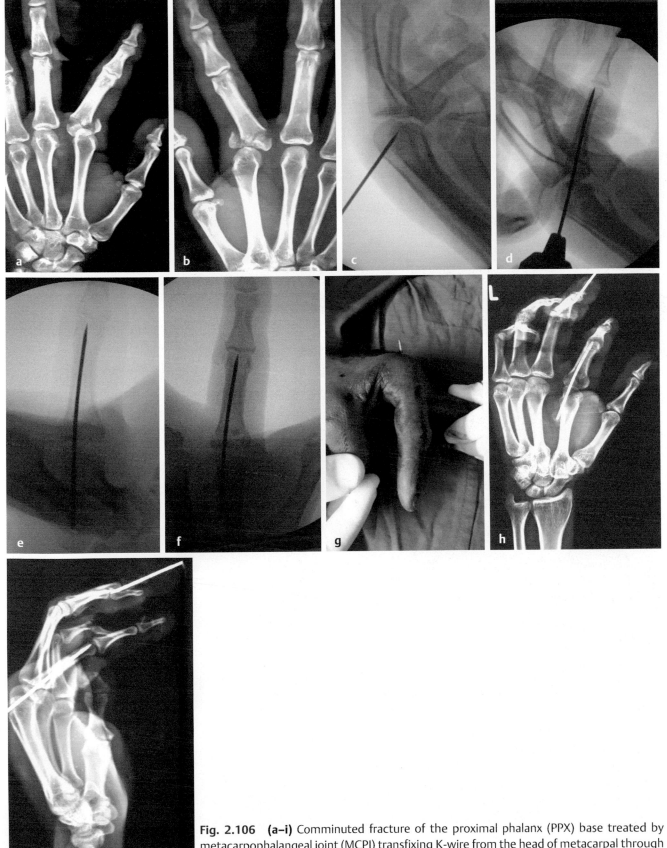

Fig. 2.106 (a–i) Comminuted fracture of the proximal phalanx (PPX) base treated by metacarpophalangeal joint (MCPJ) transfixing K-wire from the head of metacarpal through the MCPJ and PPX in 70-degree flexion.

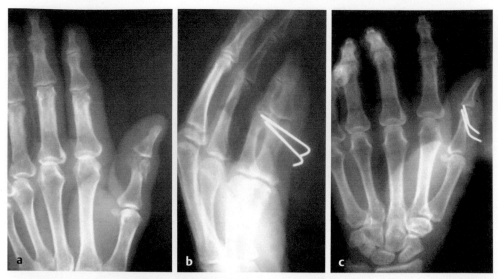

Fig. 2.107 **(a–c)** Unicondylar fracture head of the proximal phalanx (PPX) transfixed with two side-to-side K-wires.

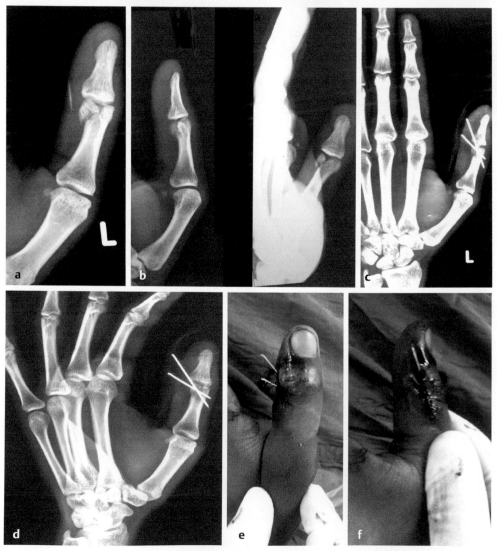

Fig. 2.108 **(a–f)** Unicondylar fracture head of the proximal phalanx (PPX) transfixed with two K-wires in divergent fashion.

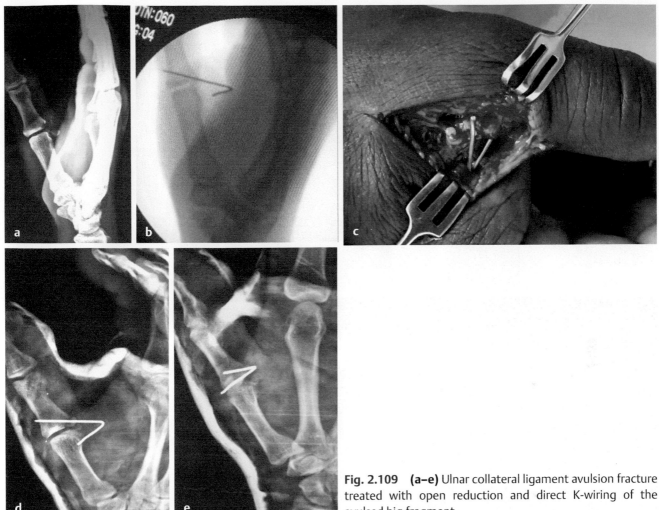

Fig. 2.109 **(a–e)** Ulnar collateral ligament avulsion fracture treated with open reduction and direct K-wiring of the avulsed big fragment.

from the DPX tip to PPX shaft maintaining the reduction and alignment for 4 weeks followed by removal and gentle mobilization with night splint for another 6 weeks. Mild angulatory deformity may appear later without much functional issue and patient needs to be warned (**Fig. 2.111a–f**).

Proximal Phalanx Shaft Fracture of Thumb

There are two methods of K-wiring this type of fracture.

The first method is desirable to treat with single intramedullary K-wire from DPX tip with IPJ transfixation in neutral position and through the PPX fracture, parking the tip at the base. This method is technically easy with less operating time, less radiation, and least complication, other than theoretical risk of damaging the articular cartilage in IPJ.

The other method is two crossed K-wires starting from the PPX base aimed for intramedullary distal fragment fixation. The rotation was aligned by flexing the thumb at the MCPJ in AP radiographic view and fixation was achieved as shown in **Fig. 2.112a, b**. Here the only problem is that dorsoulnar K-wire may impale on the extensor tendon on flexion movement of the thumb as the tracking of this tendon is more toward the ulnar side of the joint.

Comminuted Proximal Phalanx Shaft Fracture with Intra-Articular Extension Thumb (Fig. 2.113a–e)

Single intramedullary thick K-wire was used utilizing the ligamentotaxis principle. Distraction at MCPJ is obvious on entering the hard subchondral bone of metacarpal head.

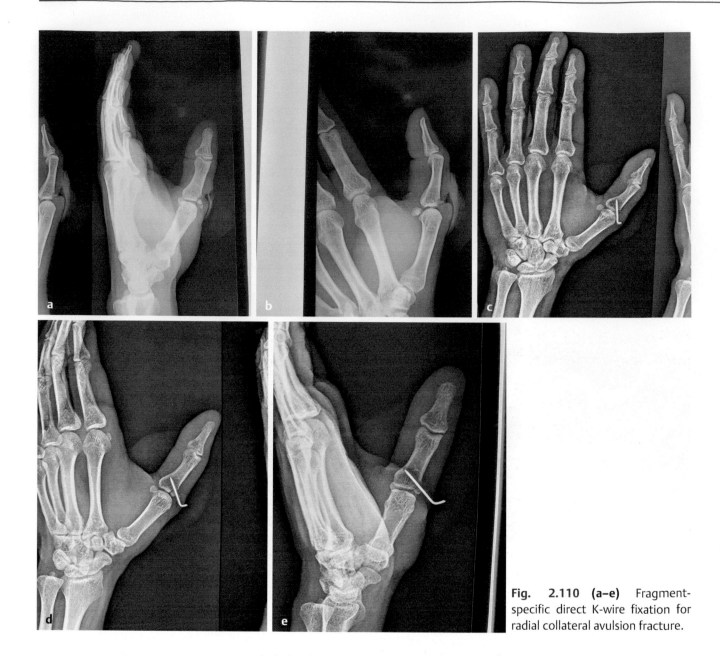

Fig. 2.110 (a–e) Fragment-specific direct K-wire fixation for radial collateral avulsion fracture.

Proximal Phalanx Comminuted Intra-Articular Fracture Shaft and Base of Thumb (Fig. 2.114a–h)

Single intramedullary K-wire in distraction mode parked at metatarsal head maintaining length and alignment.

Partial Intra-Articular Fracture Proximal Phalanx Thumb (Fig. 2.115a–h)

Using the ligamentotaxis principle, single intramedullary K-wire was passed from the DPX tip and parked in distraction mode on the head of metacarpal. IPJ transfixation in straight neutral position and MCPJ transfixation was done in 30-degree flexion to get a good purchase as in full extension it was going eccentric and missing the metacarpal head. Only problem here was the initial K-wire direction in the medullary canal was eccentric and not centered to the joint. Here the entry point was again changed to redirect. Most important message here is to use the thinnest possible K-wire because with thick K-wire the preformed tract cannot be changed again to redirect.

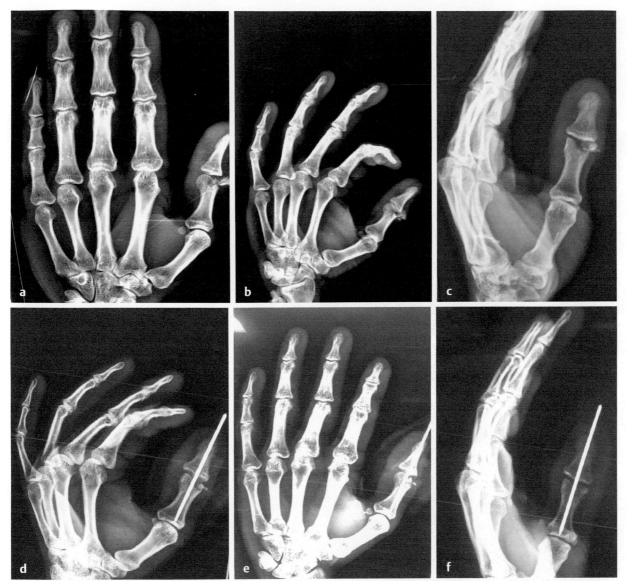

Fig. 2.111   (a–f) Open unicondylar fracture proximal phalanx (PPX) with flimsy attachment was excised and joint stabilized with intramedullary K-wire from the distal phalanx (DPX) to PPX.

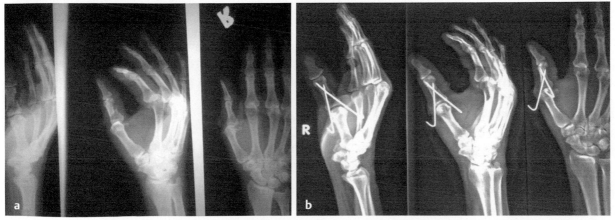

Fig. 2.112   (a, b) Two intramedullary cross K-wires from the proximal phalanx (PPX) base was done to transfix a thumb fracture.

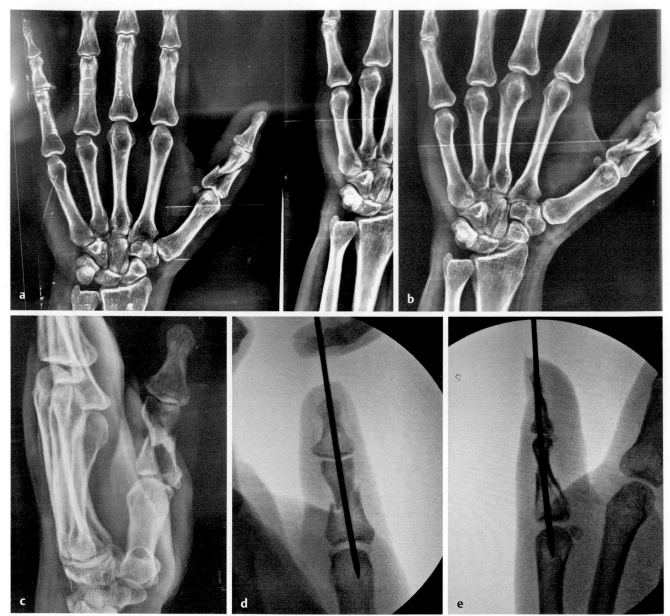

Fig. 2.113 (a–e) Comminuted intra-articular fracture proximal phalanx (PPX) thumb treated with intramedullary ligamentotaxis K-wiring.

Partial Intra-Articular Fracture Base of Proximal Phalanx Thumb (Fig. 2.116a–f)

An oblique fracture in the volar ulnar aspect of PPX with displacement was reduced with pointed reduction clamp. The orientation of the fracture and three-dimensional assessment of the fracture fragment is necessary for proper placement of K-wire. Direct transfixation K-wires were passed to secure the fragment. These wires were removed at the end of 3 to 4 weeks.

Comminuted Fracture Base of Proximal Phalanx of Thumb (Fig. 2.117a–j)

Case Scenario 1

With thumb traction and direct compression over the fracture site, a single thick K-wire snug fix at the isthmus of DPX was passed from DPX tip, and IPJ in extension and through PPX. Maintaining the traction and reduction of the fragments, the wire was transfixed across the

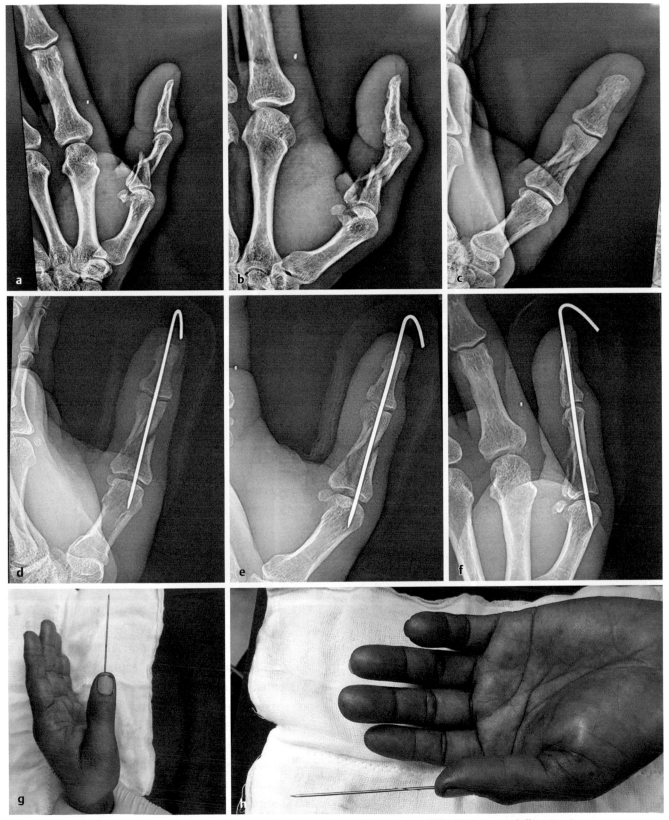

Fig. 2.114   (a–h) Comminuted shaft with intra-articular fracture of thumb treated with intramedullary K-wire.

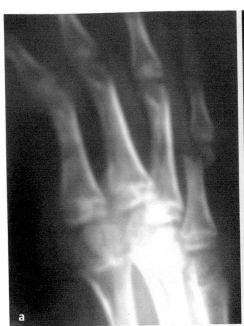
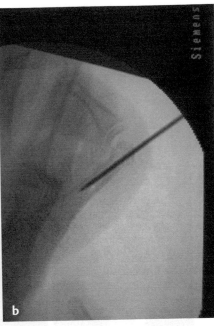

Fig. 2.122 (a, b) Small head fragment in a child reduced and fixed with direct K-wire through the proximal phalanx (PPX) head, which is not the normal way.

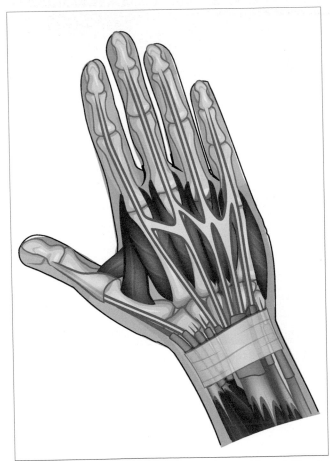

Fig. 2.123   Anatomy of extensor tendon and its relation to metacarpophalangeal joint (MCPJ).

palmar aspect (**Fig. 2.125**). The spike jetting out dorsally is clearly visible in the true lateral view. The superficial and deep transverse palmar ligament attached at the neck level gets taut on flexion of all fingers, aiding the reduction of the central metacarpals (2 & 3) but not the border digits (1, 2, & 5). On flexion the central metacarpals are pulled out of length and rotation gets corrected (**Fig. 2.126a–c**). Flexing all the fingers at the MCPJ maintains the length of the shortened third and fourth metacarpal shaft fractures because of the concertina effect of tight intermetacarpal ligament at the level of metacarpal neck. Long spiral fractures may cause gross shortening and require additional traction and pointed reduction clamp to get the spiral matched for obtaining the length.

After passing the retrograde K-wire through distal fragment from the metacarpal head and negotiating in to the proximal fragment medullary canal, the final rotational control of fracture is achieved by flexing all fingers at the MCPJ to almost 90 degrees and applying direct dorsal pressure at the apex of the deformed midshaft of metacarpal. By flexing the MCPJ, the PPX base pushes the metacarpal head dorsally correcting the dorsal angulation, and by relaxing the long flexors tendons and lumbricals, the deforming force is neutralized. Another

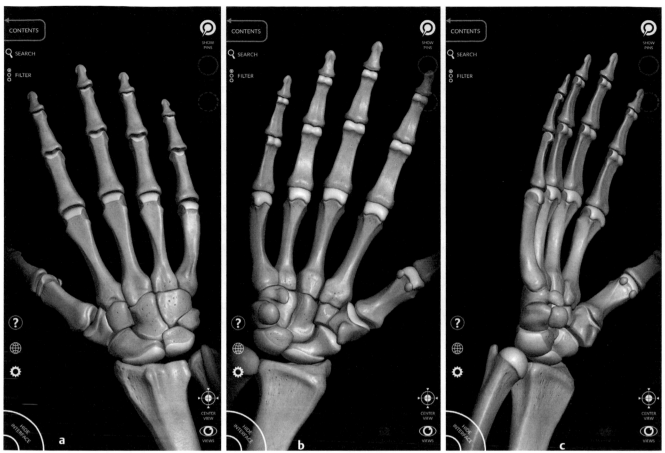

Fig. 2.124 **(a–c)** Anatomy showing the predominant articular cartilage of the distal and volar aspect of metacarpal head.

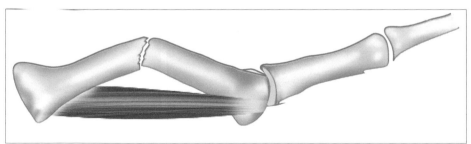

Fig. 2.125 Dorsal angulation of the metacarpal fractured fragments due to pull of the intraossei and lumbricals.

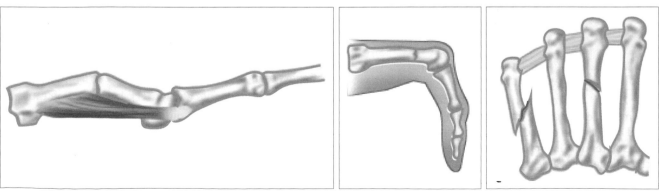

Fig. 2.126 **(a–c)** Taut transverse metacarpal ligament aiding the length and rotation correction on flexion of fingers relaxing the intrinsics.

joint holding in traction and abduction with direct pressure to correct the dorsal angulation. This reduction was checked in all positions in C-arm image picture (**Fig. 2.142a–f**).

Too much comminution of the base of first metacarpal can cause gross shortening and displacement. In this case, K-wire was passed from the intact base of first

metacarpal into the base of second metacarpal in order to maintain the height and angulation, keeping the fracture indirectly reduced (**Fig. 2.143a–d**).

Another method advocated is oblique skeletal traction for comminuted fracture of thumb metacarpal base—Thoren traction. A 1.5-mm K-wire is drilled obliquely through the proximal metacarpal shaft and it

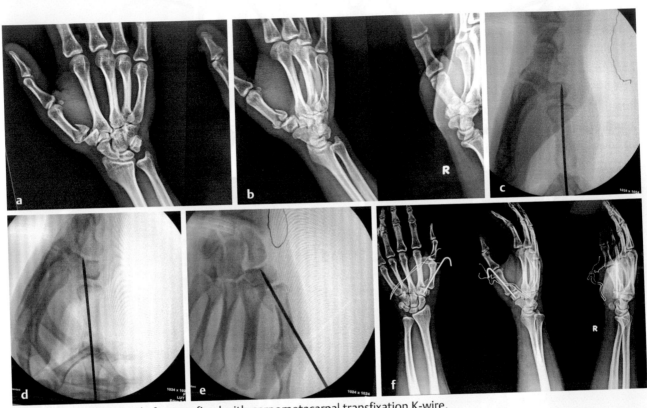

Fig. 2.142 **(a–f)** Rolando fracture fixed with carpometacarpal transfixation K-wire.

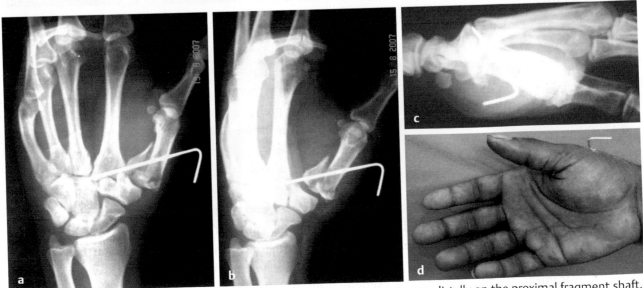

Fig. 2.143 **(a–d)** More comminution at the base needs the K-wire to start more distally on the proximal fragment shaft.

exits distally through the web space. The pin is crimped proximally and distal traction is applied through a banjo outrigger. This technique effectively counteracts both the shortening and varus angulation (**Fig. 2.144**).

Base of Fifth Metacarpal Fracture

This fracture usually results in dorsal displacement with dorsal angulation which is fully appreciated in the oblique- and lateral-view X-ray. Failure to correct this will result in loss of grip strength. This fracture was reduced with axial traction of little finger with PIPJ flexed and direct pressure over the site of angulation. First transverse K-wire was inserted 1 cm above the fracture site from medial to lateral cortex of the fifth metacarpal slightly in dorsal direction considering the transverse palmar arch. keeping the fracture reduced the K-wire was advanced in to the fourth metacarpal. In case the fourth metacarpal is not palpable with the wire one can manipulate its position by pushing down or pulling up to get double cortex fixation. Four cortex feel of piercing with K-wire is mandatory for a stable fixation. One must insert directly perpendicular to the shaft under C-arm scan control with 10-degree dorsal tilt as the metacarpals are arranged like a dome. Another transverse K-wire was added at the neck level of metacarpal for additional angular/rotational stability and fixation.

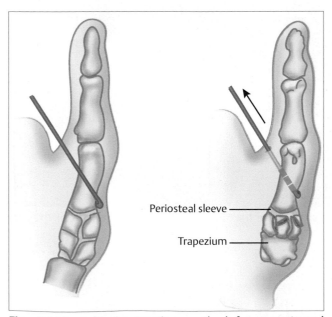

Fig. 2.144 A K-wire traction method for comminuted metacarpal base fracture.

The displaced fifth metacarpal base was reduced indirectly and transfixed to the fourth metacarpal by a transverse K-wire, as shown in **Fig. 2.145a–f**. This wire was inserted 1 cm away from the fracture site and not too far. The abductor digiti minimi muscle was pushed down palmarward before entering with K-wire to prevent tethering. The dorsal displacement was reduced by direct pressure and one should have feel of four cortices while drilling (two cortex of fifth metacarpal and two cortex of fourth metacarpal). Intramedullary K-wire may not give good purchase as the proximal fragment (base of the metacarpal) was too small.

Another case of fracture base of the fifth metacarpal with angulation and shortening. This was reduced and fixed with two transverse K-wires from the distal fragment to the fourth metacarpal shaft maintaining the length and alignment (**Fig. 2.146a–i** and **Video 2.4**).

Fifth Metacarpal Base Comminuted Intra-Articular Fracture

Shortening with dorsal shift is the major problem with this type of fracture. This comminuted fracture was reduced by traction and ligamentotaxis principle. The reduced fracture in traction was maintained in length by transfixing the shaft of fifth to fourth metacarpal by two transverse K-wires. The dorsal displacement or subluxation is common in this type of injury, and this was always reduced by direct dorsal pressure first K-wire starting at the base of fifth metacarpal to transfix to fourth metacarpal and second at the level of midshaft as shown in **Fig. 2.147a–d**.

Another scenario of the base and proximal shaft of the fifth metacarpal comminuted fracture with intra-articular extension is shown in **Fig. 2.148a–d**. Here to maintain the length, alignment, and rotation, intermetacarpal K-wires were done. First with traction the dorsal angulation at fracture site was corrected and an intermetacarpal wire just a centimeter distal to the fracture was passed. The wire must enter perpendicular to the shaft passing transversely through the two cortices of the fifth and the fourth metacarpal considering the palmar arch. The feel of piercing each cortex (near and far cortex of each bone) while drilling is important like the resistance and giving way for adequate fixation. Once the reduction is maintained, next transverse K-wire

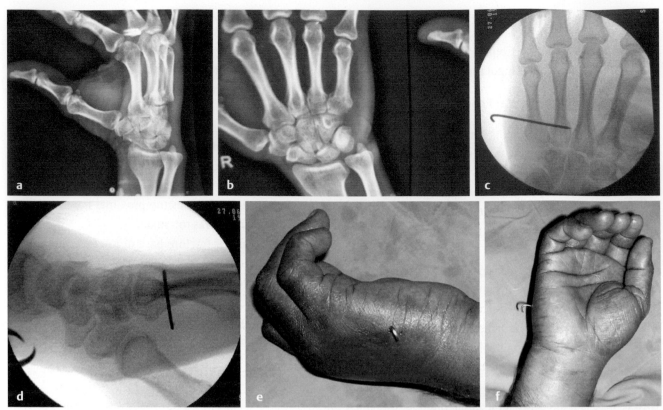

Fig. 2.145 **(a–f)** A transverse K-wire from the base of fifth metacarpal (MC) was inserted in reduced position to the fourth MC by feeling four-cortex fixation.

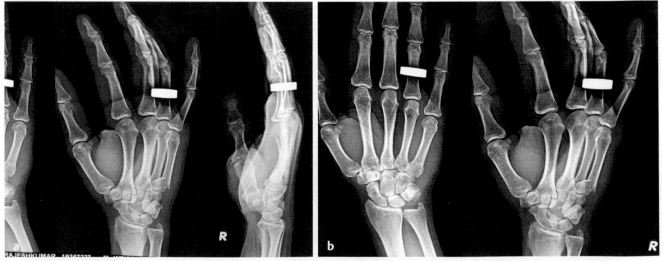

Fig. 2.146 **(a–b)** Two transverse indirect K-wire fixations to maintain the fracture reduction and alignment of the fifth metacarpal base and fracture. *(Continued)*

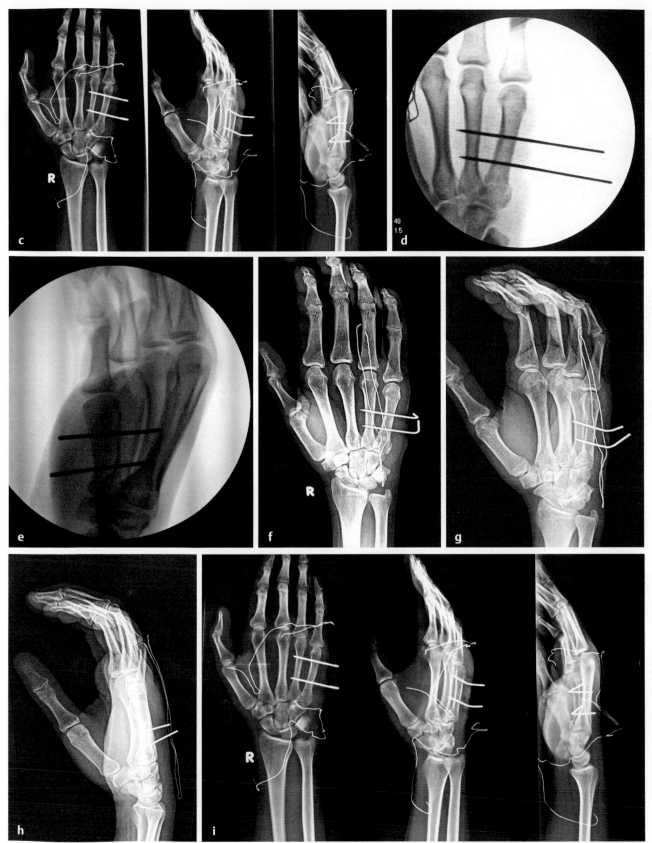

Fig. 2.146 (*Continued*) **(c–i)** Two transverse indirect K-wire fixations to maintain the fracture reduction and alignment of the fifth metacarpal base and fracture.

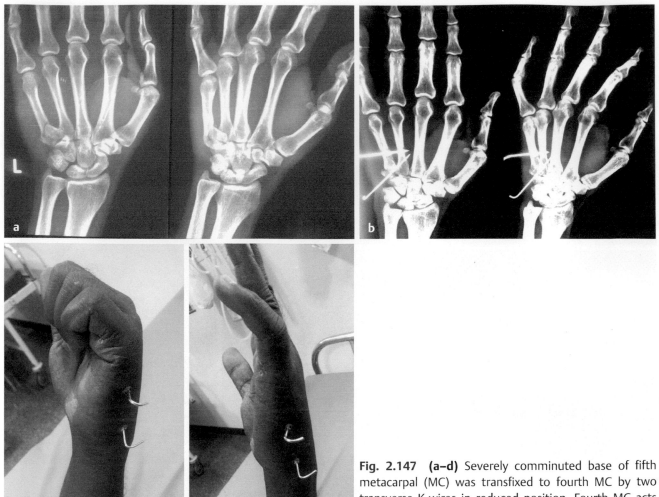

Fig. 2.147 (a–d) Severely comminuted base of fifth metacarpal (MC) was transfixed to fourth MC by two transverse K-wires in reduced position. Fourth MC acts like an internal splint to hold the fracture.

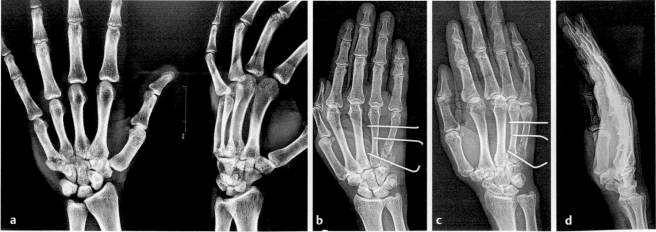

Fig. 2.148 (a–d) Comminuted shaft and base of fifth metacarpal fracture warranting two indirect transverse K-wire fixation into fourth metacarpal and another direct transverse K-wire at the base.

was done 2 to 3 cm distal to the first wire in the same manner. Here one more transverse K-wire was added to the metacarpal base to align the articular fragments together.

Fifth Metacarpal Base Fracture Fixed with Intramedullary K-Wire

This fracture demonstrates marked dorsal angulation at the site of fracture with dorsal displacement. The fracture was reduced with traction to little finger in flexed position and by direct pressure over the dorsum. Both anteroposterior and lateral views of a retrograde intramedullary K-wire passing from the head in to the center of the medullary canal are important. Only then it can be transfixed to the hamate for a better hold as shown in **Fig. 2.149a–g**.

Sometimes if this fails to transfix in to the carpometacarpal joint a horizontal intermetacarpal K-wire may be necessary just distal to the fracture to correct dorsal displacement.

Extra-Articular Fracture Base of the First Metacarpal of Thumb

Case Scenario 1

This can be treated either like a Bennett fracture dislocation with adjacent joint transfixation oblique K-wire (**Fig. 2.150a, b**).

Case Scenario 2

If the fracture is more proximal it can be transfixed in a retrograde intramedullary K-wire from the metacarpal head in to the trapeziometacarpal joint (**Fig. 2.151a–f**).

Case Scenario 3

This fracture behaves in a similar manner to Bennett fracture subluxation. The fracture was reduced by traction on the thumb and by direct pressure over the dorsal angulation. A 2-mm K-wire was passed 1 cm distal to the fracture along the line of metacarpal in true anteroposterior view directing toward trapezium at an angle of 60 degrees to the metacarpal. This wire would transfix the fracture maintaining the reduction and further inserted in to trapezium transfixing the trapeziometacarpal joint.

The reduction was confirmed in various oblique and lateral views (**Fig. 2.152a–e**).

Metacarpal Neck Fractures

Management of all metacarpal neck fractures with K-wire should follow the sequence of steps elaborated as below after perfect closed reduction by Jahss maneuver (**Fig. 2.153**) which involves flexing MCP 90 degrees and PIPJ 90 degrees. A dorsal force is applied to metacarpal head with axial load on PPX and counterpressure on the metacarpal shaft palmarward. Stretching of collateral ligaments of MCPJ also aids in perfect reduction.

Case Scenario 1

Second metacarpal neck fracture with displacement (**Fig. 2.154a–w**). A 1.8- or 2-mm K-wire is selected depending on the isthmus diameter. The sharp tip of smooth K-wire was cut so that it does not catch the cortex while negotiating through the medullary canal. A gentle bend of 20 degrees was given at 4 mm from the blunt-tip K-wire. A 2.5 mm drill bit was used to create a pilot hole at the metacarpal base by pushing the first dorsal interosseous muscle away as shown in **Fig. 2.154**. In index finger it was done at the dorsolateral cortex at the metaphyseal flare with the help of C-arm image intensifier. Initially the drill was started perpendicular to the bone and then gradually tilted to 60 degrees and more parallel to the shaft. The hole can be enlarged in more parallel direction to the shaft, so that the bent-tip K-wire can be passed through it easily. The K-wire was negotiated in to the medullary canal by turning the wire with tip pointing toward the medullary canal and convex surface of the bend abutting the opposite cortex. With to-and-fro rotary movement with axial force using the cannulated plier, the wire was advanced further to the fracture site. The reduction was obtained by axial pull of the finger in flexed position and the tip of the wire was advanced in the head fragment. Once the reduction was perfect, the rotation of the K-wire can bring the convex tip buttressing the head along the long axis and the tip was parked subchondrally with gentle hammering of the K-wire. This will prevent back out of K-wire or loss of reduction. Adequate reduction and positioning of the wire was checked before bending the K-wire.

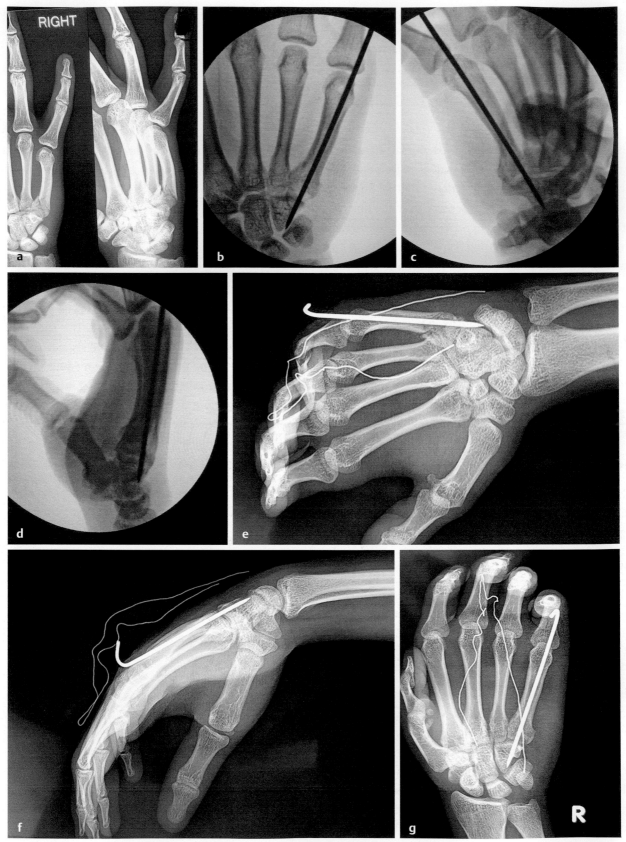

Fig. 2.149 (a–g) Fifth metacarpal base fracture with dorsal angulation corrected with intramedullary retrograde K-wiring and parking on the hamate.

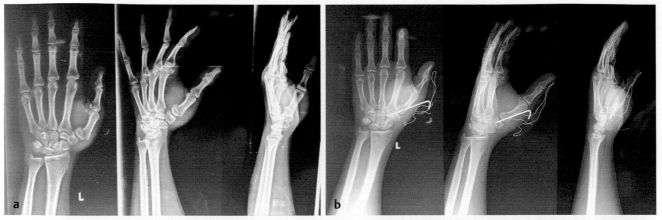

Fig. 2.150   (a, b) Juxta-articular fracture base of first metacarpal fixed with transfixation K-wire like in Bennett fracture.

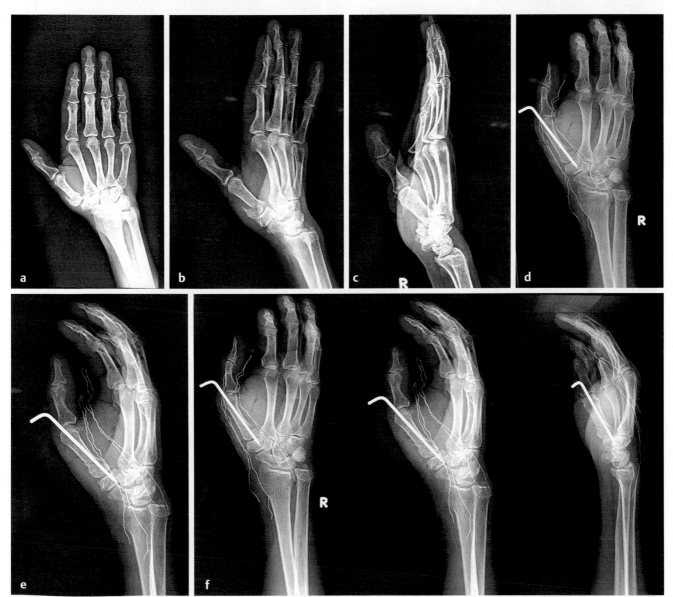

Fig. 2.151   (a–f) Fracture in the distal third metacarpal fixed with retrograde intramedullary K-wire from the metacarpal head into trapezium.

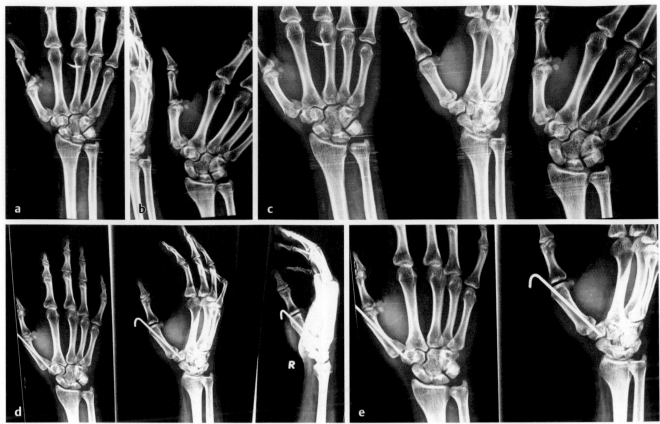

Fig. 2.152 **(a–e)** Extra-articular fracture base of first metacarpal fixed with joint transfixation K-wire.

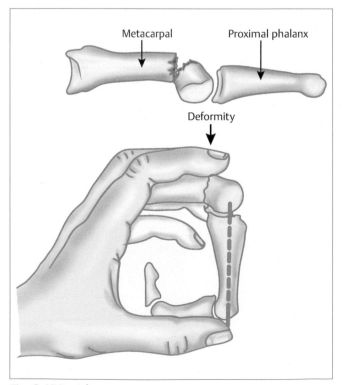

Fig. 2.153 Jahss maneuver.

Case Scenario 2

Fifth metacarpal neck fracture (Boxer fracture) (**Fig. 2.155a–d**). Palmar tilt with angulation of more than 40 degrees with extension lag on active extension is an indication for correction of the deformity. Cosmetically, the knuckle prominence will come back with correction of the deformity, with restoration of good grip strength. X-ray shows distal third, fifth metacarpal fracture extending up to the neck. This was corrected by closed antegrade intramedullary K-wire passed from the base of the dorsum of fifth metacarpal. At first a 2.5-mm drill bit was used to start the entry point at the base of the fifth metacarpal on the dorsoulnar aspect. The drill entry was started perpendicular to make an impression on the bone and then gently angulated along the line of the shaft to make an oblique entry hole. A straight 1.8-mm thick K-wire with blunt tip and slight bent at the tip (15 degrees) was negotiated through the entry point into the shaft of the metacarpal, checking the position in the medullary canal,

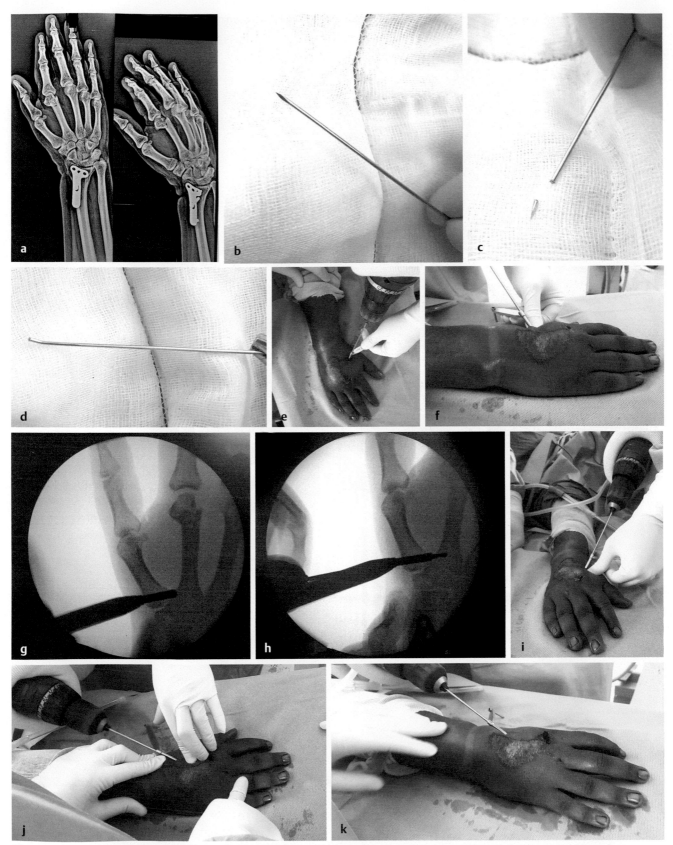

Fig. 2.154 **(a–k)** Technique of antegrade intramedullary K-wiring for second metacarpal neck fracture. *(Continued)*

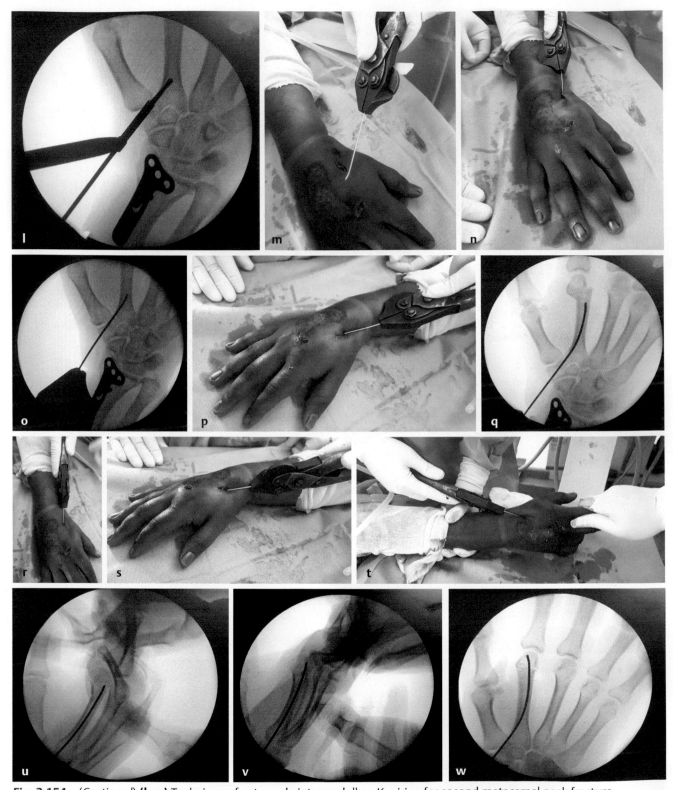

Fig. 2.154 (*Continued*) **(l–w)** Technique of antegrade intramedullary K-wiring for second metacarpal neck fracture.

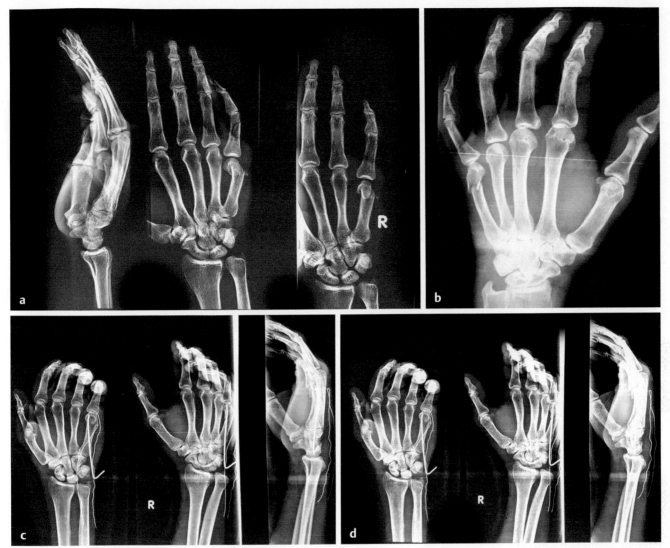

Fig. 2.155   (a–d) Antegrade intramedullary K-wire for fifth metacarpal neck fracture.

in both anteroposterior and lateral C-arm image. A cannulated plier holding the K-wire was used to advance by axial force with to-and-fro oscillating movement gently, so that it does not abut the cortex and stop (one should not drill to prevent false track). After passing through the fracture site, angulation was reduced by two methods: (1) By direct manual pressure and hyper extension of the little finger to correct flexion. (2) By Jahss maneuver: Flexing the MCPJ relaxes the intrinsics and tightens the ligaments. The PPX can be used to reduce the fracture with upward axial thrust to push the metacarpal head in to extension and metacarpal shaft with opposite downward pressure. Wire was placed up to subchondral

bone to hold the reduction. Always check the position of K-wire by anteroposterior, lateral, and oblique views to make sure the tip has not come out through fracture line.

From day one full finger range of movement exercises was started without any discomfort for the patient. The K-wire was removed at the end of 4 weeks.

Late presentation up to 3 weeks sometimes requires intrafocal K-wire manipulation and reduction.

Case Scenario 3 (Fig. 2.156 a–f)

Fracture neck and shaft of fifth metacarpal fixed with intramedullary antegrade K-wire from base of fifth metacarpal.

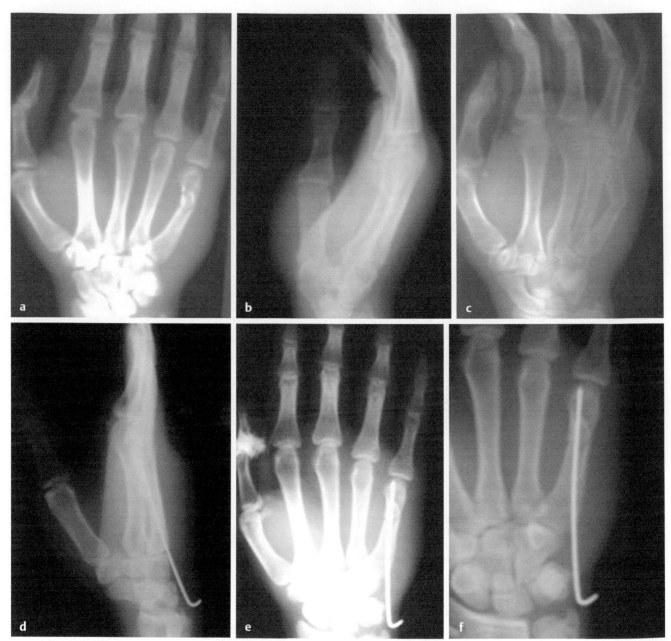

Fig. 2.156 (a–f) Fifth metacarpal neck fracture was fixed by passing a prebent blunt-tip K-wire after making an entry with a 2.5mm drill at the base of metacarpal (MC). Once entered into the medullary canal, only plier is used to negotiate the wire distally, fracture reduced, and wire parked subchondrally with slight impaction to have a good hold.

Case Scenario 4

Fifth neck of metacarpal fracture with angulation in a 10-year-old child (**Fig. 2.157a–c**). A similar procedure to adult fracture was done. The fracture was reduced by closed manipulation and antegrade K-wire was passed from the base of the fifth metacarpal.

Case Scenario 5

Fracture Neck of Fifth Metacarpal with Volar Tilt (**Fig. 2.158 a, b**). An antegrade K-wiring from the base of the fifth metacarpal was done. The fracture was reduced anatomically and fixed with the tip of the wire engaging subchondrally.

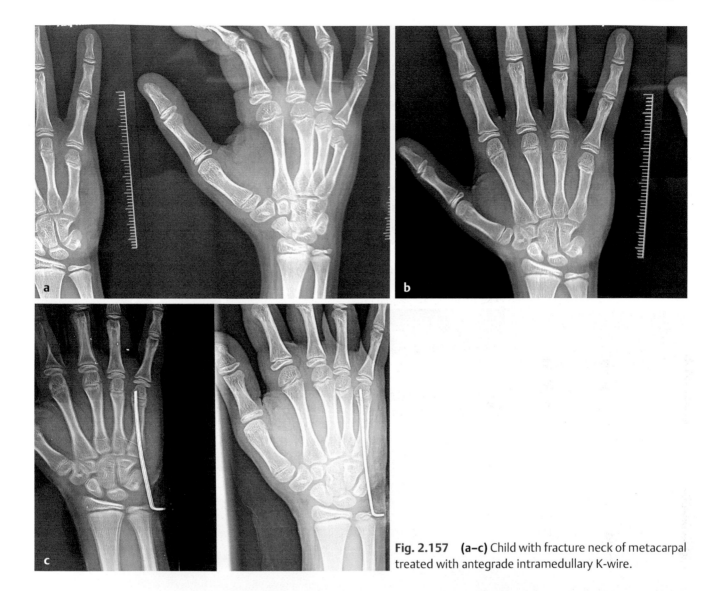

Fig. 2.157 **(a–c)** Child with fracture neck of metacarpal treated with antegrade intramedullary K-wire.

Fig. 2.158 **(a, b)** Reduction with Jahss maneuver and intramedullary K-wire fixation.

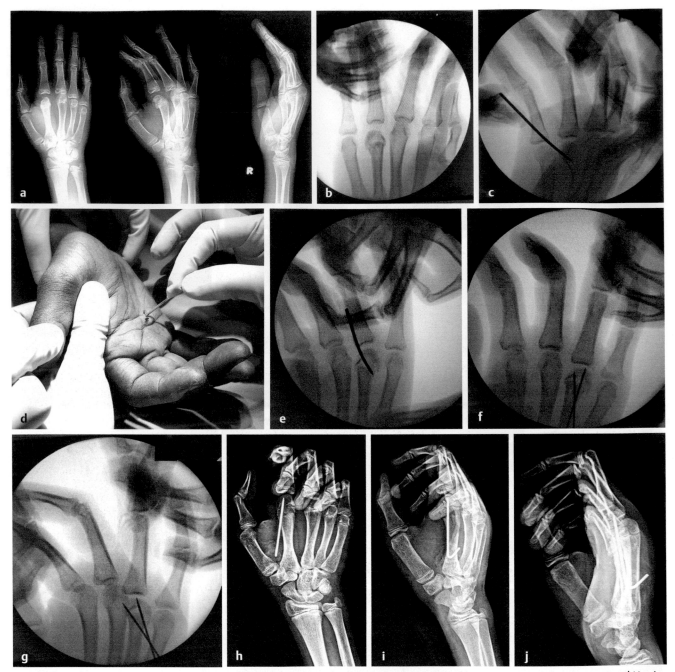

Fig. 2.161 **(a–j)** Second metacarpal physeal fracture with volar displacement reduced by percutaneous maneuver and K-wire transfixation.

Long Oblique Fracture Head of Fifth Metacarpal (Fig. 2.164a–e)

An antegrade K-wire from the base of the fifth metacarpal was passed. The wire was negotiated through the fracture holding in good position with a cannulated plier and parking the tip of the wire subchondrally buttressing the head fragment.

Comminuted Long Spiral Fourth Metacarpal Fracture Neck and Shaft (Fig. 2.165a–d)

This is a longitudinal comminuted fracture starting from head to middle third shaft of metacarpal that was collapsed with loss of height and rotated. Here a prebent tip K-wire of 2-mm thickness was passed from the metacarpal base. Predrilling the entry point at the base with

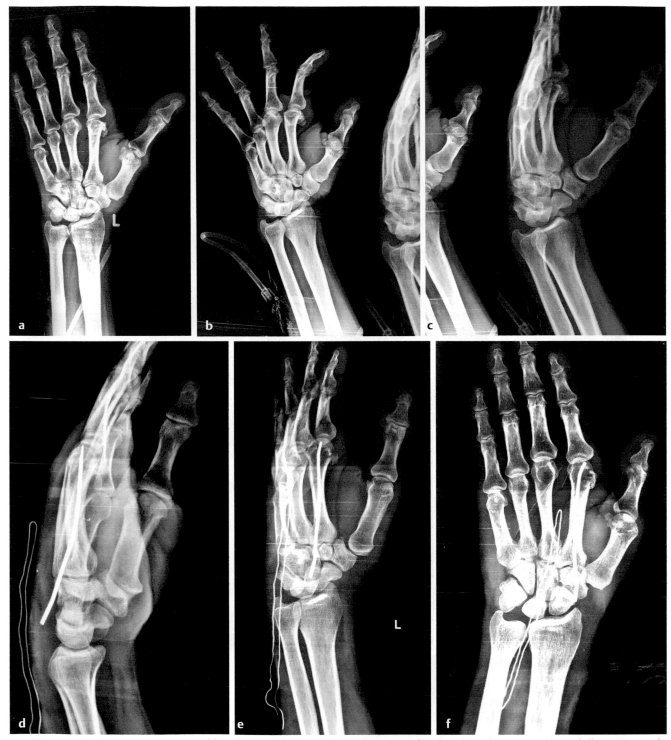

Fig. 2.162 **(a–f)** Second metacarpal head fracture with volar displacement fixed with prebent tip intramedullary antegrade K-wire.

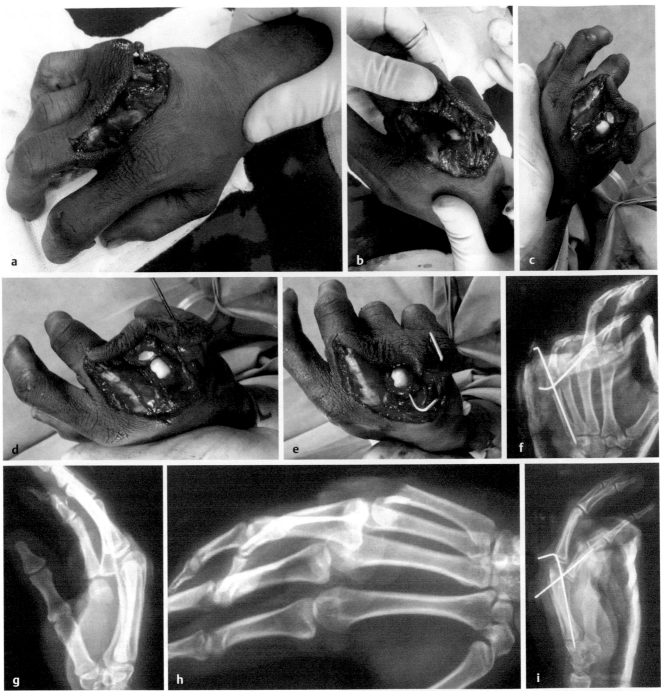

Fig. 2.174 **(a–i)** Crush injury of the hand with loss of tissues and bone stabilized with intramedullary K-wire for fifth metacarpal (MC) neck fracture. Open fourth metacarpophalangeal joint (MCPJ) with bone loss stabilized with fourth MCPJ joint transfixation wire from the head of fourth MC, keeping MCPJ at 70-degree flexion and wire entering proximal phalanx (PPX) intramedullary.

Hand Deformity

Adduction Deformity of Thumb

Adduction deformity or Z-deformity of thumb was caused by Volkmann ischemic contracture of the forearm and hand in an 11-year-old child. This occurred due to supracondylar fracture treated 4 years ago.

This deformity was corrected by adequate adductor release, capsular contracture release, and trapeziectomy. The corrected position was maintained by transfixing the K-wire of scaphoid and first metacarpal in good abduction in an ante/retrograde manner. K-wire was inserted through the metacarpal base to come out distally and then from distal to proximal into scaphoid in the desired position, as shown in **Fig. 2.175a–g**.

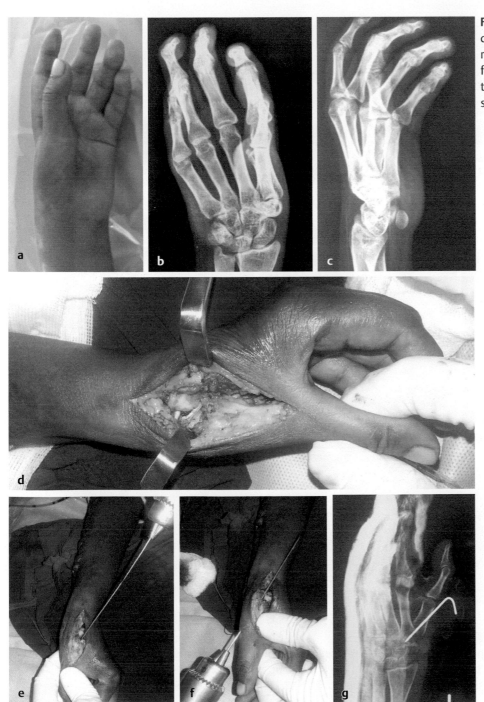

Fig. 2.175 (a–g) Adduction deformity correction by soft tissue release, trapeziectomy, and K-wire fixation in corrected position transfixing first metacarpal to scaphoid.

Volkmann Ischemic Contracture

Extreme claw hand deformity and wrist flexion contracture from severe Volkmann ischemic contracture had deformity correction to achieve functional position for better hand function. Child had lengthening of long flexors of fingers and wrist, capsular contracture release of the MCPJ, and long extensors lengthening. The corrected claw hand deformity (hyperextension at MCPJ) was flexed to 70 degrees and transfixed with K-wire passing from the metacarpal neck into MCPJ and medullary canal of the PPX, as shown in **Fig. 2.176a–g**. One K-wire got missed out from the PPX, but served the purpose like a splint. Checking the position of K-wire in different views of image intensifier could have avoided this problem. These K-wires were retained for 4 weeks and served as an internal splint.

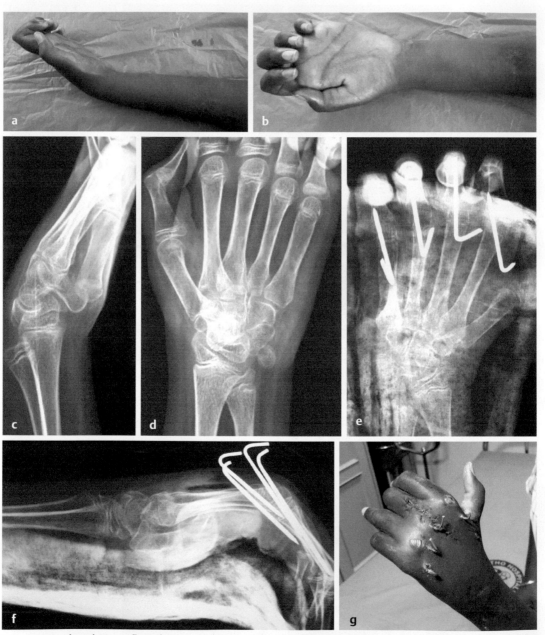

Fig. 2.176 **(a–g)** Hyperflexed wrist and severe claw hand from extreme hyperextension corrected by soft tissue release. Metacarpophalangeal joint (MCPJ) flexed up to 70 degrees and maintained by joint transfixation K-wire passing from dorsum of metacarpal (MC) head aiming to the center of medullary canal of flexed proximal phalanx (PPX).

3 Wrist

Scaphoid Fracture

Acute Scaphoid Fracture

The proximal pole and waist fracture of the scaphoid can be anatomically reduced by closed means and fixed with percutaneous K-wires. The distal palmar tuberosity of the scaphoid is palpated as shown in **Fig. 3.1**. This is located immediately proximal to the thenar eminence and immediately radial to the flexor carpi radialis tendon. The opposite hand is used to move the patient's hand/wrist unit into flexion–extension and radioulnar deviation. If one is palpating the distal pole of scaphoid, this small bony lump will move, demonstrating that it is a part of the carpus and not the radius. More importantly, the distal pole will become prominent palmarly with radial deviation as the scaphoid rotates into flexion.

The distal pole of scaphoid on the volar aspect of the wrist is palpated; K-wire sized 1.5 mm is passed from the volar radial aspect of the scaphoid, aiming into the proximal pole at a 60-degree angle to the forearm axis, in anteroposterior (AP) and lateral views, after anatomical reduction of the scaphoid fracture. The entry point of the K-wire must skirt the trapezium so that it is slightly ulnar to the outer border of the scaphotrapezial joint and aimed toward the proximal pole, through the waist.

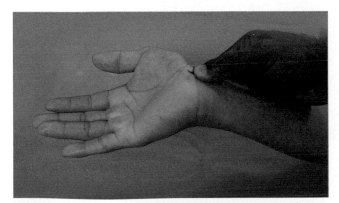

Fig. 3.1 Palpation of distal tuberosity of the scaphoid.

The tip of the wire is placed subchondrally to maintain the length. In a displaced fracture, K-wire entering the distal pole can be used as a joystick to manipulate and correct the volar flexion and ulnar deviation of the fragment. Another K-wire was passed in perfect position as described earlier by maintaining the reduction with the K-wire used as a joystick. Sometimes two K-wires are passed in a similar fashion, parallel to each other to give a rotational stability. These percutaneous wires are left outside and a scaphoid cast is applied for 6 weeks, until the fracture heals in **Fig. 3.2a–e**. Another example of scaphoid fracture is illustrated in **Fig. 3.3a–d**.

Distal Radius Fracture with Scaphoid Fracture

Fig. 3.4a–h shows an example of distal radius fracture first fixed; and then scaphoid is manipulated on a stable platform, reduced and fixed with two K-wires.

Cannulated Cancellous Screw Fixation

Insertion of K-wire after reduction of the fracture scaphoid has been described earlier. If compression at the fracture site is necessary, then a cannulated cancellous screw or Herbert screw or headless AO screw (AO Foundation, Davos, Switzerland) can be used as shown in **Fig. 3.5a–e**. In this case, the placement of K-wire in the scaphoid must be in the center for proper positioning of the screw.

Scaphoid Nonunion

It is a case of long-standing scaphoid nonunion that has led to a painful wrist with radioscaphoid and midcarpal arthritis. Because of the preservation of radiolunate joint, it was managed with scaphoid excision with capitolunate triquetrohamate fusion (four-corner fusion) (**Fig. 3.6a–c**).

Open surgical procedure was performed with removal of the cartilage and subchondral bone from intercarpal

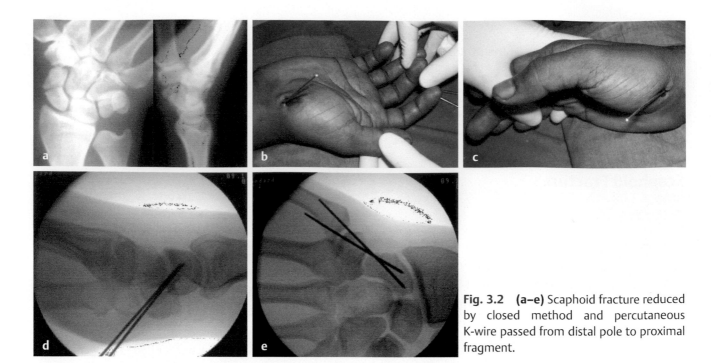

Fig. 3.2 (a–e) Scaphoid fracture reduced by closed method and percutaneous K-wire passed from distal pole to proximal fragment.

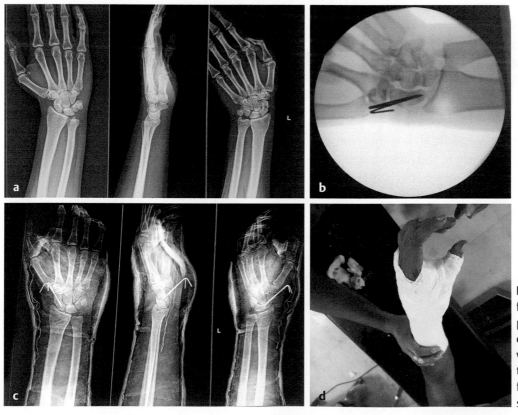

Fig. 3.3 (a–d) Scaphoid fracture at waist with displacement and foreshortening due to volar flexion was reduced and fixed with two percutaneous K-wires for rotational stability and scaphoid cast was given.

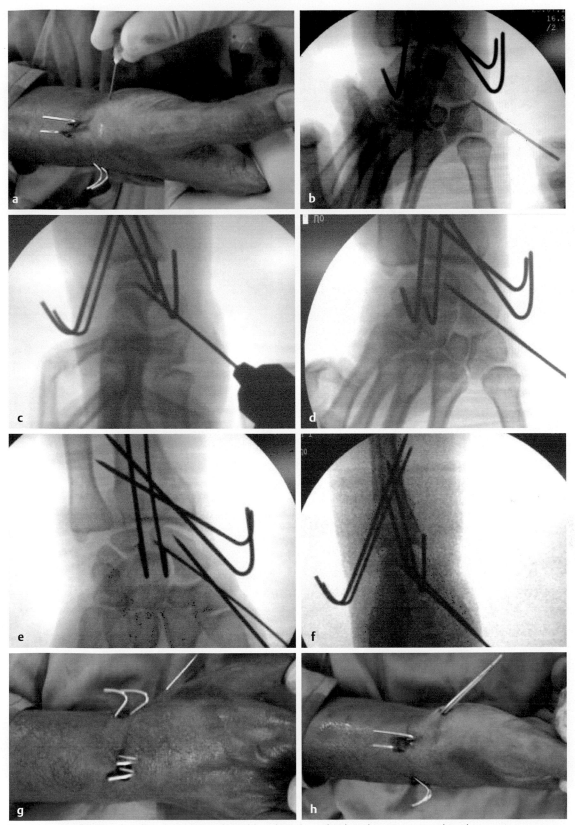

Fig. 3.4 **(a–h)** Distal radius fracture reduced by closed method and K-wire passed in the routine manner. Scaphoid fracture was reduced and K-wire fixation was done from the distal to proximal fragment.

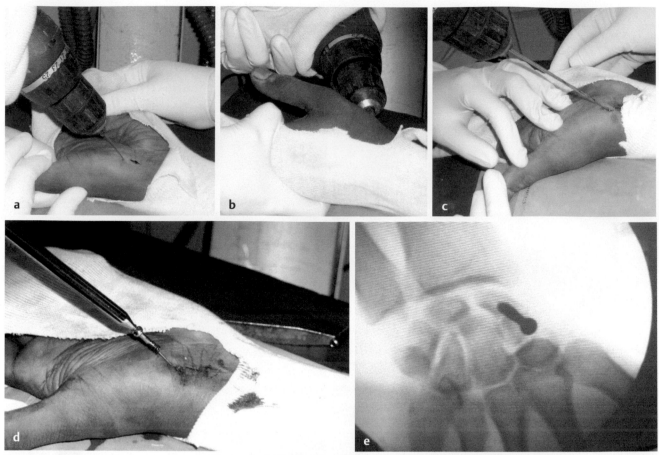

Fig. 3.5 **(a–e)** The K-wire used to transfix scaphoid fracture can be substituted with cannulated screw system.

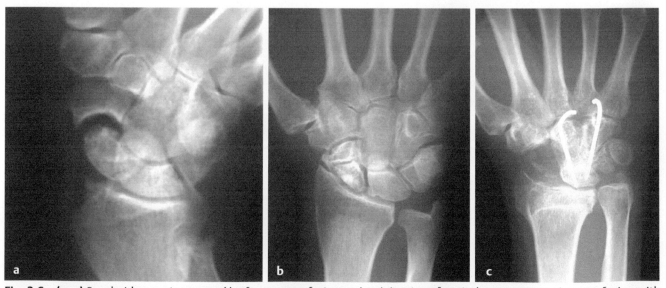

Fig. 3.6 **(a–c)** Scaphoid nonunion treated by four-corner fusion and stabilization of capitolunate triquetrohamate fusion with grafts and K-wires.

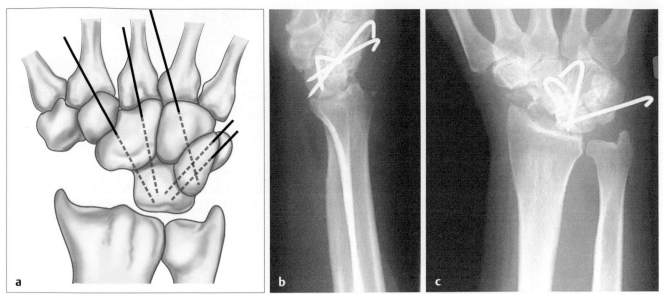

Fig. 3.7 **(a–c)** K-wire passed through capitolunate, triquetrolunate, and hamatolunate for four-corner fusion.

articulations and bone graft laid in the gaps. K-wire was passed through capitolunate, triquetrolunate, and hamatolunate under fluoroscopy control as shown in **Fig. 3.7a–c**. Below-elbow plaster of Paris (POP) cast was given for 3 months until radiological evidence of fusion was seen.

Scapholunate Dissociation Injury (Fig. 3.8a–i)

Scapholunate dissociation injury results in dorsal intercalated segmental instability (DISI) deformity with typical increase in scapholunate distance in AP X-ray view (Terry Thomas sign). The lunate dorsally tilted was corrected to neutral position by volar flexion of the wrist. In this position, a transosseous K-wire was passed from the base of radial styloid in lateral to medial direction pointing the trajectory toward the center of lunate. Once the lunate was fixed, the palmar flexed scaphoid was brought to the normal palmar tilt of 45 degrees by gentle dorsiflexion of the wrist. The scaphoid lunate gap becomes normal and scaphoid was anchored in this position by another K-wire starting from the radial styloid process distal to the previous wire, toward the scaphoid in lateral to medial direction. As the wire was holding the scaphoid eccentrically, another K-wire in similar fashion was inserted for a better hold and purchase. Maintaining

the relationship of scaphoid and lunate in this position in acute injury will make the ligaments to heal properly. A scaphoid cast in tumbler holding position was given. The below-elbow cast and K-wires were removed at the end of 6 weeks.

Radial Styloid Fracture

Radius styloid fracture, which was innocent looking after 1 week, showed scapholunate dissociation with positive Terry Thomas sign (widening of space between scaphoid and lunate). This was immediately taken up for closed manipulation and reduction of DISI deformity by passing the first K-wire from the lateral aspect of radius to lunate thereby transfixing the bone in neutral position. Similar K-wire was passed from radius to scaphoid maintaining the scapholunate angle and correcting the dissociation (**Fig. 3.9a–i**).

Radial Styloid Fracture with Scapholunate Dissociation (Fig. 3.10a–e)

All radial styloid fracture must be carefully studied to rule out scapholunate injuries of varying degrees. In this case, the radial styloid tip fracture was associated with scapholunate dissociation. Terry Thomas sign was positive with foreshortened scaphoid indicating palmar flexion. This was reduced by closed means by two transverse K-wire applied across scaphoid and lunate in reduced

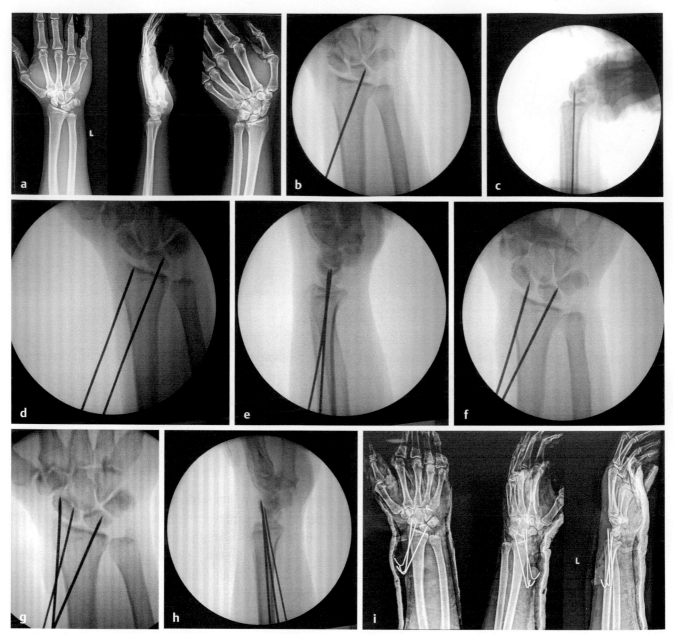

Fig. 3.8 **(a–i)** Scapholunate dissociation injury.

position. A below-elbow cast was given for 6 weeks and then mobilized the hand joints. Final good alignment of carpal bones was seen at 8 weeks postinjury.

Radial Styloid Fracture with Scapholunate Dissociation (Fig. 3.11)

The radial styloid fracture was reduced, dorsal tilt with subluxation of radiocarpal joint was corrected, and the styloid fragment was fixed with a 2 mm K-wire. The scapholunate dissociation got corrected partially, revealing the DISI deformity. This was corrected by putting transfixing K-wire, introduced from the radius into the lunate bone in corrected radiolunate alignment as shown in Sometimes, two K-wires were used if the purchase was marginal on the lunate. These wires were left for 6 weeks until the fracture and ligaments mended properly.

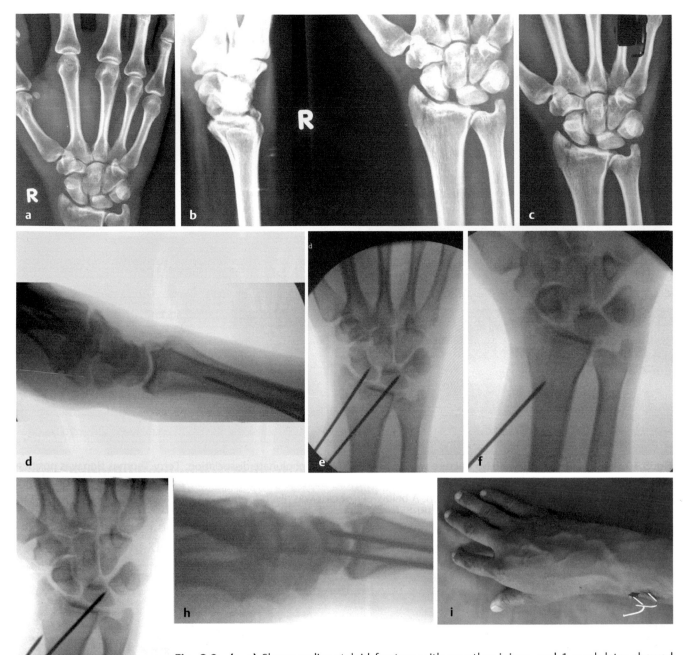

Fig. 3.9 **(a–c)** Shows radius styloid fracture with no other injury, and 1 week later showed obvious scapholunate dissociation. **(d–i)** Demonstrates the method of correction of dorsal intercalated segmental instability (DISI) deformity and K-wire insertion.

Perilunate Dislocation (Fig. 3.12)

Patient had a fall from motor bike and sustained perilunate dislocation. The Gilula's arc was broken indicating an abnormal proximal row alignment. The scaphoid was rotated, and the lunate no longer articulates with capitate. This was reduced by closed method. Once reduced, check for scaphoid fracture, which is not uncommon. Percutaneous K-wire fixation was done to prevent loss of reduction and later scapholunate dissociation, and to enhance the healing of intrinsic ligaments.

A K-wire was passed from the radial styloid laterally into the lunate in neutral position without any volar or dorsal tilt. Once radiolunate alignment was restored, the scaphoid was aligned to lunate in lateral view of 45 to 60 degrees. The scaphoid was secured in the desired

styloid in comparison with ulnar styloid tip. Then the dorsal and radial displacement is corrected by palmar flexion and ulnar deviation. After anatomical reduction, the position is maintained by placing the hand on a rolled towel with palmar flexion and ulnar deviation (**Fig. 3.22a, b**) and secured with at least three percutaneous K-wires.

- Palpate the Lister tubercle over the radial aspect of the dorsal distal radius. First incision is made dorsal and distal to the Lister tubercle. Artery forceps is used to spread the soft tissues; K-wire is introduced on the Lister tubercle in 45-degree obliquity aiming the volar cortex of the proximal fragment in the long axis of radius. If the entry is slightly ulnar to the Lister tubercle, it may injure the extensor pollicis tendon. After insertion of the first K-wire, make sure that image intensifier shows good reduction in both AP and lateral views. One should proceed to the next step only if this is correct in height of the radius, alignment, normal palmar tilt, no translation, or radial tilt. One cannot and should not manipulate the fragment after putting the first wire, as it is unlikely to change and will only bend the existing K-wire. If the reduction is unacceptable, one should remove the first K-wire, remanipulate, and start fresh again.

- Second incision is made over the styloid process, 0.5 cm distal to the radial styloid process tip; artery forceps is introduced to split the soft tissues. By blunt dissection, bone is reached so that one can avoid injury to the superficial sensory branch of the radial nerve and the tendons of the first dorsal compartment. The K-wire is introduced from the tip of the radial styloid, centering anteroposteriorly in the lateral view as a superimposed shadow over the bony contour of lunate. From here, K-wire is angled 60 degrees to the radial shaft, transfixing fracture by piercing the ulnar aspect of the radius.

- Third wire is passed to fix the lunate fossa fragment (dorsoulnar rim) by incising the skin nearly 0.5 cm distal to the wrist joint line (third incision). By blunt dissection with artery forceps, the bone is reached and usually it is between the fourth and fifth extensor compartments. K-wire is introduced from the dorsal margin of the lunate fossa fragment at 45-degree angle parallel to the adjacent dorsal wire and transfixed into the volar aspect of the radius as shown in **Fig. 3.23a, b**.

Distal radius fracture fixed with percutaneous K-wiring using three-wire technique in a classical manner is shown in **Fig. 3.24a–e** and **Video 3.1**. Distal radius fracture fixed with percutaneous K-wiring and demonstrating finger movements is illustrated in **Fig. 3.25a–d**.

Kapandji described a technique where by two or three K-wires were inserted into the fracture site (intrafocal pinning) to directly manipulate and correct the distal fracture fragment into the desired position. Once the reduction was achieved, the wires were advanced into the proximal fragment. The pins do not fix the distal fragment but rather buttress it in place. In the original description, patients were not immobilized postoperatively. Kapandji originally advocated this technique for

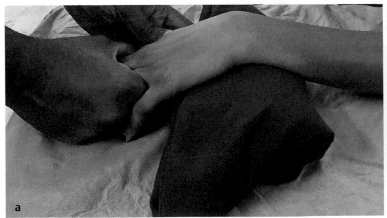
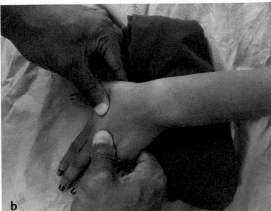

Fig. 3.22 **(a, b)** Using a small towel under the wrist, one can easily reduce the dorsally displaced fracture by volar flexion and ulnar deviation force maintaining traction as shown.

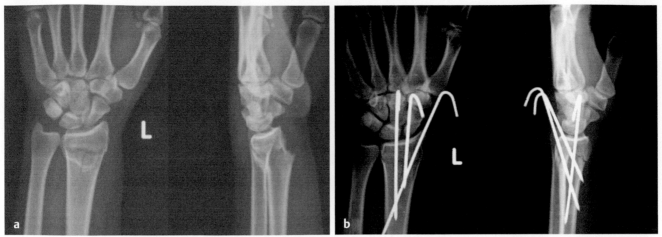

Fig. 3.23 **(a, b)** Typical Colles fracture reduced and fixed with a dorsal K-wire through Lister tubercle, another wire from the radial styloid to proximal fragment, and third wire from lunate fossa fragment.

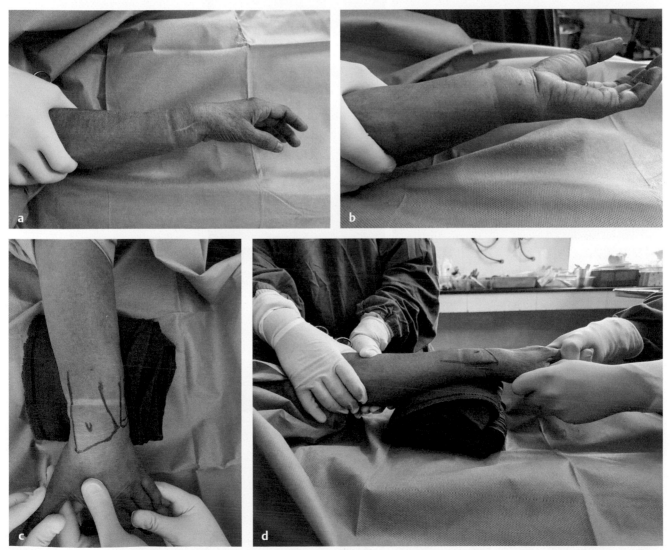

Fig. 3.24 **(a–d)** Step by step demonstration of closed reduction technique with percutaneous K-wire fixation of distal end radius fracture. *(Continued)*

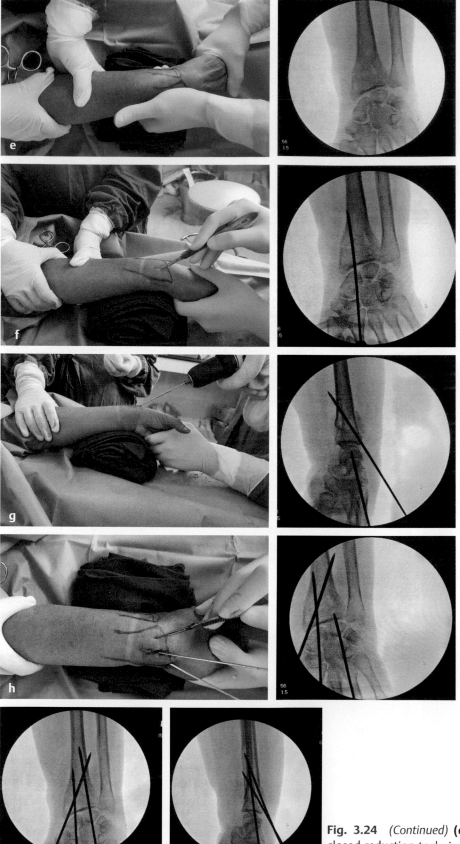

Fig. 3.24 *(Continued)* **(e–i)** Step by step demonstration of closed reduction technique with percutaneous K-wire fixation of distal end radius fracture.

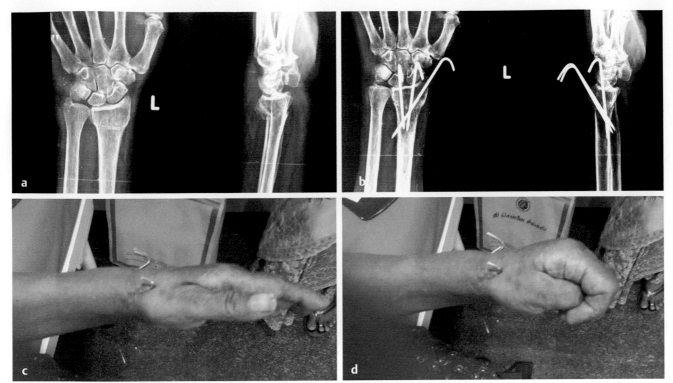

Fig. 3.25 (a–d) Postoperative distal radius K-wire fixation demonstrating active finger flexion making a fist comfortably.

younger patients, whose fractures were only minimally comminuted. It was contraindicated in patients with osteoporotic bone or severe comminuted and in fracture with intra-articular extension. Intrafocal pinning by itself does not provide rigid fixation and loss of reduction is quite possible which is a major disadvantage (**Fig. 3.26a–f**).

Fracture Distal Radius and Ulna in an Elderly Patient (Fig. 3.27a–c)

Closed manipulation and reduction of distal radius is done and secured with three percutaneous K-wire in the conventional manner. The distal ulna fracture at metadiaphyseal junction required intramedullary K-wire through the ulnar styloid with which the dorsal tilt was corrected and passed intramedullary in to the ulna shaft. An above-elbow slab was given for ulnar fracture immobilization to prevent rotational force.

Tips and Pearls for Distal Radius Fracture

- The fixation on the volar side of proximal fragment (far cortex) can be very close to the fracture,

resulting in break of the cortex and loss of fixation. Both the dorsal wires should not transfix into the volar cortex of the radius in the same horizontal line as it may break the volar cortex leading on to loss of fixation. The volar fixing wire must be 2 cm away from the fracture site. Short-segment fixation close to the fracture may lead to loss of reduction on mobilization of the wrist, as shown in **Fig. 3.28a–c**.

- The K-wire passed from the distal to proximal fragment sometimes may not transfix the proximal fragment and it may slide intramedullary. This may lead to early wire pullout and loosening, loss of height, and fixation, though it may look good intraoperatively. Definitely one should aim for bicortical K-wire fixation. If the wire slips intramedullary because of the oblique entry of the K-wire, there are maneuvers to bite the far cortex which are mentioned as follows:
  - Changing the entry point and angulating more acutely toward the volar cortex.
  - Withdrawing the K-wire going to the medullary canal up to the entry point and drilling it slowly

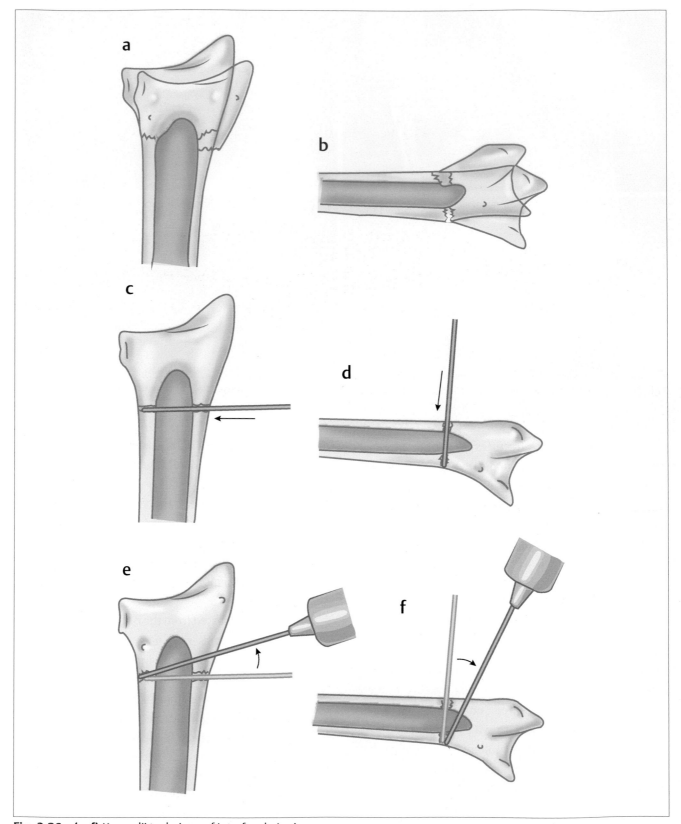

Fig. 3.26 **(a–f)** Kapandji technique of intrafocal pinning.

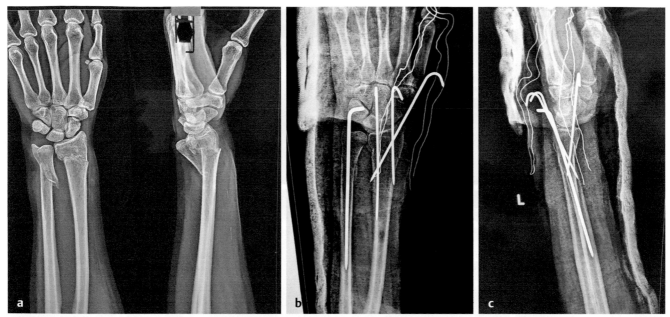

Fig. 3.27 **(a–c)** Distal radius and ulna fracture where distal radius fixed with three percutaneous K-wire and ulna fracture with intramedullary K-wire.

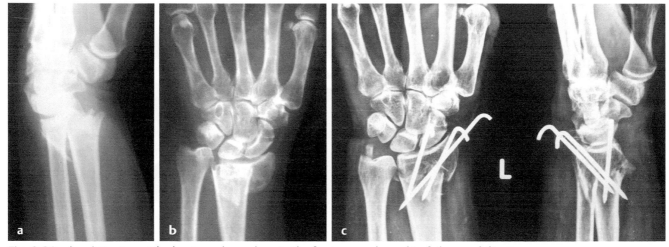

Fig. 3.28 **(a–c)** K-wires with short purchase close to the fracture are bound to fail on mobilization.

with manipulation of the wire to give a bend while drilling, as shown in **Figs. 3.20** and **3.21**. On engaging the far cortex, the K-wire should not be drilled with pressure as it may slip once again into the medullary canal. Drill should be run at high speed with little axial loading.

➤ In extreme comminution of the dorsal cortex, always try to engage the K-wire in the near cortex of the intact dorsal rim for a good

purchase. Try not to enter through the fracture site of the distal fragment as this may lead to loss of reduction and dorsal tilt. **Fig. 3.29a–e** shows dorsal rim entry of K-wire with adequate long purchase in the proximal fragment.

➤ In severely comminuted osteoporotic fractures, Kapandji intrafocal technique of passing multiple K-wires straight through the fracture site with only proximal cortex fixation is not

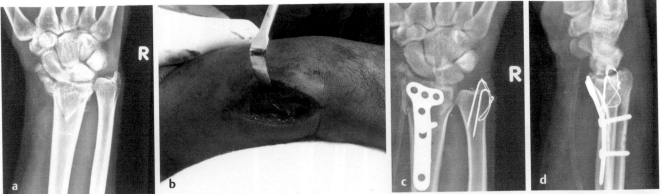

Fig. 3.41 (a–d) Comminuted distal radius fracture with ulnar styloid fracture stabilized with locking plate for radius and two K-wires with figure-of-8 tension band wire for ulnar styloid fracture.

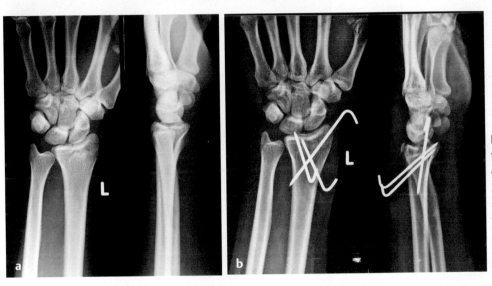

Fig. 3.42 (a, b) Three-wire technique of fixing minimally displaced volar Barton fracture, 2 dorsal K-wires passed in antiglide manner aiming toward the volar rim and another radial styloid K-wire from volar to dorsal trajectory in lateral to medial direction.

Case Scenario 1

Dorsal K-wire fixation for volar Barton fracture (**Fig. 3.43a–f**).

Case Scenario 2

Dorsal and volar radial styloid K-wire fixation for volar Barton fracture (**Fig. 3.44a–f**).

Method 2

In completely displaced fracture either by closed manipulation or sometimes percutaneous K-wire manipulation through fracture site was necessary to get the reduction; two volar and radial styloid K-wires were used. Here the forces acting were too much and only volar-routed wires can neutralize the volar tilting force. But the problem is too many structures are in the harm's way (tendons, median nerve, vessels); hence, it is not the first option. In case this needs to be done then meticulous attention at the site of K-wire entry is important to make sure by mini-incision and dissection. The indications being hemophilia, open fracture with soft tissue loss, and contamination where plating is contraindicated.

Case Scenario 3

Fig. 3.45a–p shows a patient with hemophilia of severe type with gross swelling, pain, and deformity in a 42-year-old gentleman who was right-hand dominant. Because of this bleeding disorder, there was extreme swelling with pain and skin blistering. He was initially treated with below-elbow POP slab immobilization for a

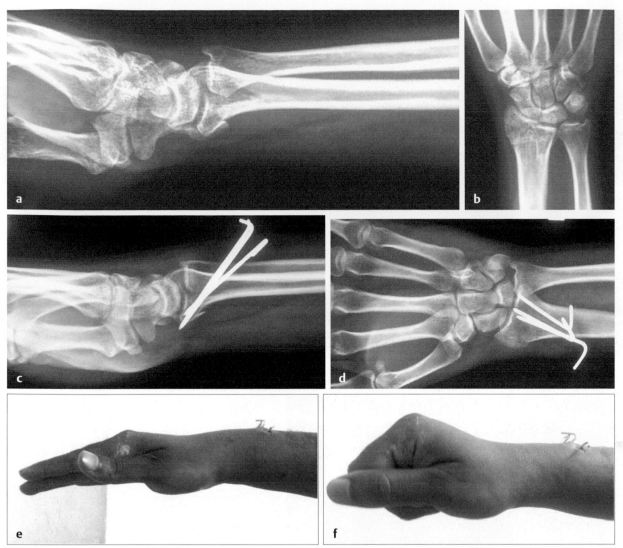

Fig. 3.43 **(a–d)** Volar Barton fracture stabilized with three dorsal K-wires with tip positioned on volar fragment in reduced position; **(e, f)** shows range of movements.

week. In the meantime, the availability of factor 8 concentrate was enquired. Patient was not very affordable to have full cover with adequate factor 8 concentrate during and after the procedure. Patient was not willing for an open procedure because of the fear factor and the cost involved. Hence a percutaneous K-wire fixation was done with perioperative factor 8 cover for a period of 24 hours. A thick K-wire was introduced through the fracture plane from volar aspect to correct the volar tilt. Another K-wire was used from radial side through the fracture plane to correct the radial tilt. First fracture transfixation K-wire was passed by holding the reduction with arm supinated. A skin nick on the volar side radial

aspect was made and an artery forceps was introduced to dissect straight to the volar rim. By this method one can avoid impaling the flexor tendons, medial nerve, and vessels. Once we are sure on the bone, a 2-mm K-wire was passed to transfix the fracture. Similarly another K-wire on the lunate fossa fragment was passed from volar side. Third wire was passed from the radial styloid volar aspect in the coronal plane to radial shaft. All three wires were holding the reduction in good position and a wrist brace was given for a period of 6 weeks. Finger, elbow, and shoulder movements were started from day one postoperative and K-wires were removed at the end of 6 weeks.

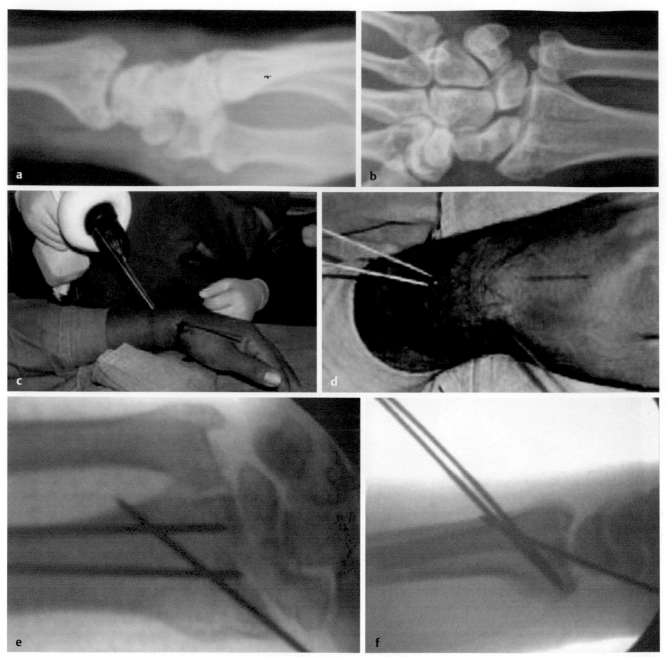

Fig. 3.44 (a–f) Volar Barton fracture with volar subluxation of the carpal bone was first reduced by a volar radial styloid K-wire in order to transfix the fragment and then two additional K-wires were introduced from the dorsal cortex to volar fragment.

Supplementary K-Wire Fixation after Volar Barton Fracture (Fig. 3.46a, b)

Percutaneous K-wire was used to correct the dorsal tilt of distal radius after performing a volar plate buttressing in volar Barton fracture. Here the radius styloid was a separate fragment which required fragment-specific fixation with K-wire.

Minimally Displaced Volar Rim Fracture Distal Radius (Fig. 3.47a–d)

Young boy sustained this injury due to a fall and presented with severe pain and localized swelling. CT scan revealed volar radial rim fracture. This was reduced by miniopen percutaneous method. A skin nick was made and artery forceps was used to dissect down to the

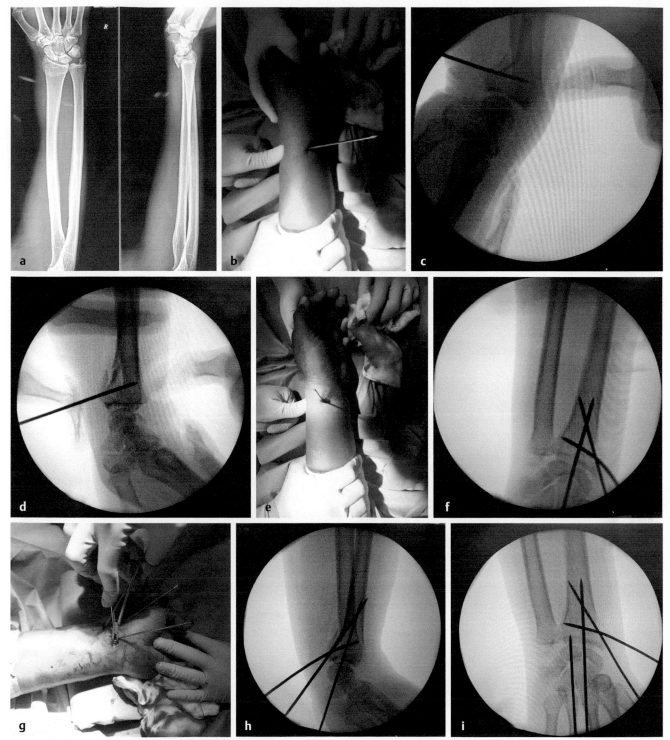

Fig. 3.45 **(a–i)** Step by step demonstration of grossly displaced volar Barton in a hemophilic patient treated with percutaneous K-wire fixation. *(Continued)*

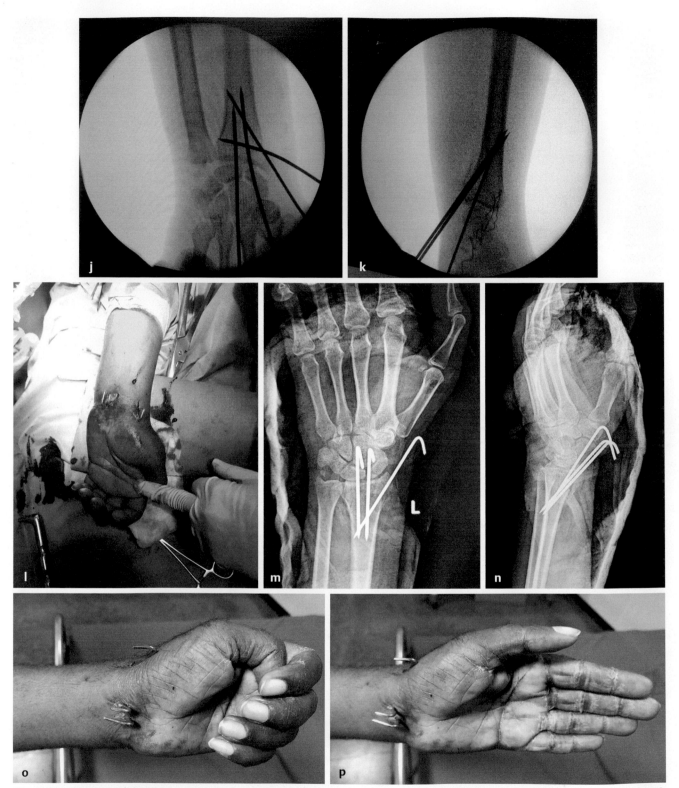

Fig. 3.45 *(Continued)* **(j–p)** Step by step demonstration of grossly displaced volar Barton in a hemophilic patient treated with percutaneous K-wire as fixation with good finger movements.

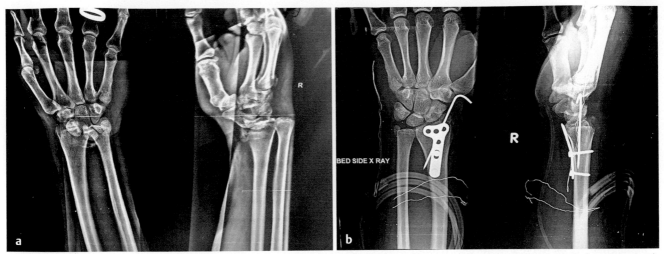

Fig. 3.46 (a, b) Buttress plating of volar Barton fracture with supplementary fixation of radial styloid separate fragment with percutaneous K-wire.

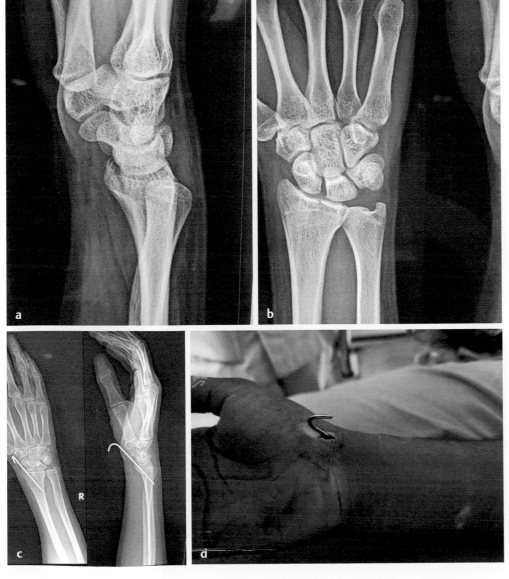

Fig. 3.47 (a–d) Miniopen percutaneous K-wire fixation for volar rim fracture.

fragment separating the tendons, vessels, and nerves. A 2.5-mm K-wire was directly placed over the fragment, and with axial pressure, the reduction was obtained. The K-wire was transfixed to opposite dorsal cortex maintaining the reduction. The wire was kept for a period of 4 weeks and wrist brace support was given.

Pediatric Distal Radius Fracture

Salter Harris Type II Distal Radius Fracture with Volar Displacement (Fig. 3.48a–d)

Fracture was reduced by traction, countertraction, and dorsiflexing the wrist. A K-wire was passed from radial styloid process at more volar aspect aiming the shaft dorsally and medially. Second K-wire was passed from the distal radial shaft midlateral aspect to the physis and epiphysis of distal radius but not piercing into the joint. One should not pass a wire from the dorsal aspect as it may pass through the fracture plane. Check for the stability of fixation by volar and dorsiflexion of the wrist under C-arm control. One should be aware of not going too volar on the radial styloid as the radial artery

is at risk. Postoperatively below-elbow plaster slab was placed in neutral position (**Fig. 3.48a–d**).

Extra-Articular Distal Radius Fracture with Dorsal Displacement and Tilt in a Child (Fig. 3.49a, b)

Extra-articular distal radius fracture was reduced by manipulation with traction, volar flexion, and ulnar deviation; K-wires were placed from styloid process and dorsal distal epiphysis into the shaft as in adult fracture fixation.

Distal Ulna Physeal Separation with Volar Displacement Distal Radius (Fig. 3.50a–g)

Complete physeal separation of distal ulna with volar tilt of distal radius fracture was treated with closed manipulation of distal radius and ulna. The ulnar epiphysis did not get reduced, warranting percutaneous K-wire to manipulate the fragment and get it reduced on distal ulna metaphysis. The reduction was maintained with above-elbow cast without any fixation.

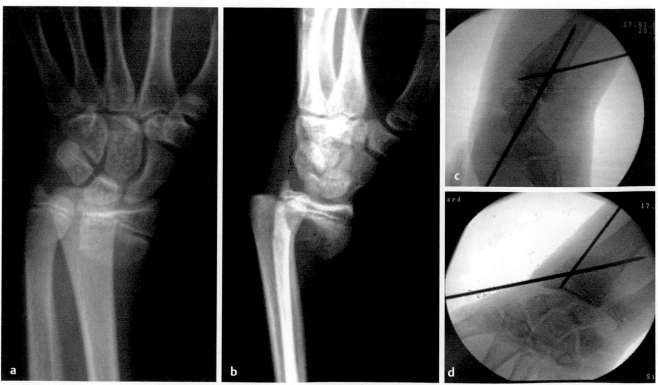

Fig. 3.48 **(a–d)** Salter Harris type II distal radius fracture stabilized with two cross transphyseal K-wires.

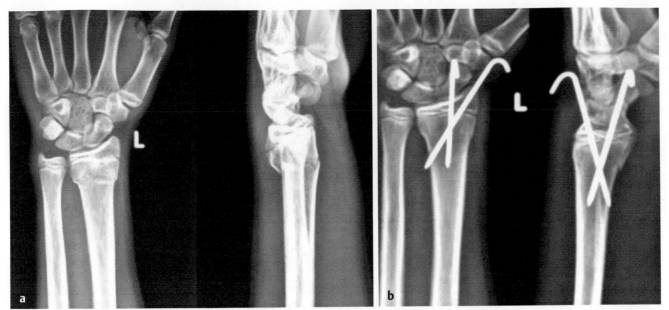

Fig. 3.49 (a, b) Immature skeleton with extra-articular distal radius fracture stabilized with two cross K-wires entering through radial styloid and dorsal K-wire through metaphysis to diaphysis.

Distal Radius Physeal Separation with Volar Displacement (Fig. 3.51a–c)

In a child with volar displacement of distal radius epiphysis due to physeal fracture was reduced by closed manipulation, dorsiflexion with direct pressure over the fragment, and the fracture was secured stable with percutaneous two smooth K-wires from radial styloid process through the physis into the metaphysis of distal radius. Here the pitfall is putting a dorsal wire which will not neutralize the volar displacement force and the trick is even the radial styloid wire is directed to the dorsomedial aspect of distal radius shaft to buttress the volar displacement force (starting from more volar radial aspect in the styloid process and directing toward the dorsal and medial shaft of radius).

Two-Weeks Old Quadratus Fracture Distal Radius and Ulna (Fig. 3.52a–g)

By closed manipulation reduction was difficult. A thick K-wire was used to negotiate through the fracture site and using it like a crowbar the distal fragment was levered on the proximal fragment to distalize and correct the angulation. Once the reduction was achieved, two cross K-wires were passed in the routine manner maintaining the reduction. An above-elbow POP cast was given for additional support and to prevent supination pronation movement. The K-wires and POP were removed at the end of 5 weeks.

Pediatric Volar Radial Displacement of Distal Radius with Distal Ulna Shaft Fracture (Fig. 3.53a, b)

This was reduced by closed method and a midlateral radial styloid wire was used to transfix the reduced fragment first. A mid-dorsal wire was also inserted through the physis transfixing the fracture. We tend to use minimum wires (two here) in pediatrics where the physis need to be crossed. Ulna fracture was reduced by closed method and an intramedullary retrograde wire through styloid process transfixing the fracture was done. An above-elbow POP slab was given for additional support and safety.

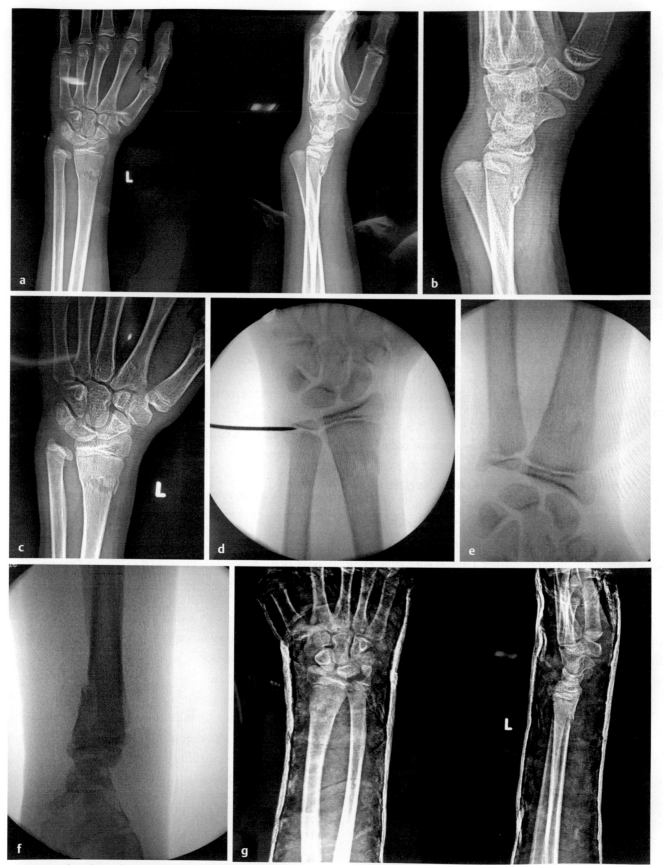

Fig. 3.50 **(a–g)** Displaced distal ulna epiphysis was relocated using percutaneous K-wire and above-elbow cast application.

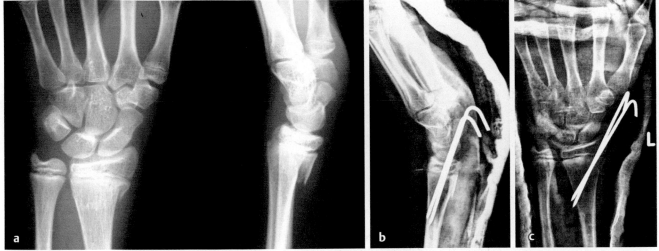

Fig. 3.51 (a–c) Salter Harris type II distal radius fracture with volar displacement treated with closed reduction and two percutaneous K-wires from radial styloid volar to dorsal trajectory in lateral to medial direction.

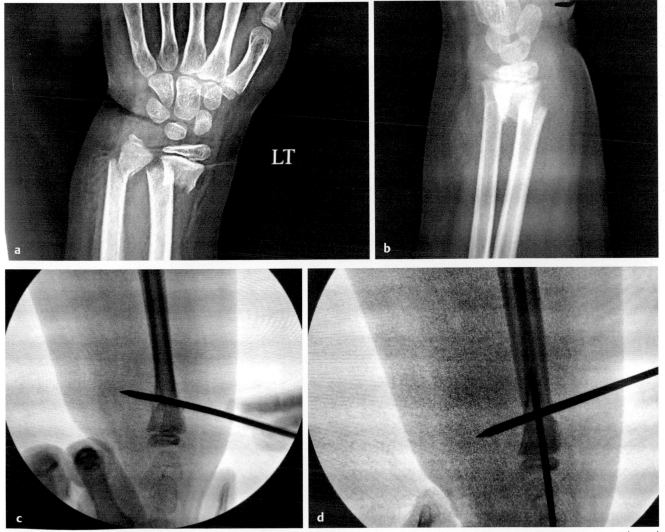

Fig. 3.52 (a–d) Delayed presentation of quadratus fracture manipulated using percutaneous K-wire as joystick and transfixation K-wire fixation done. *(Continued)*

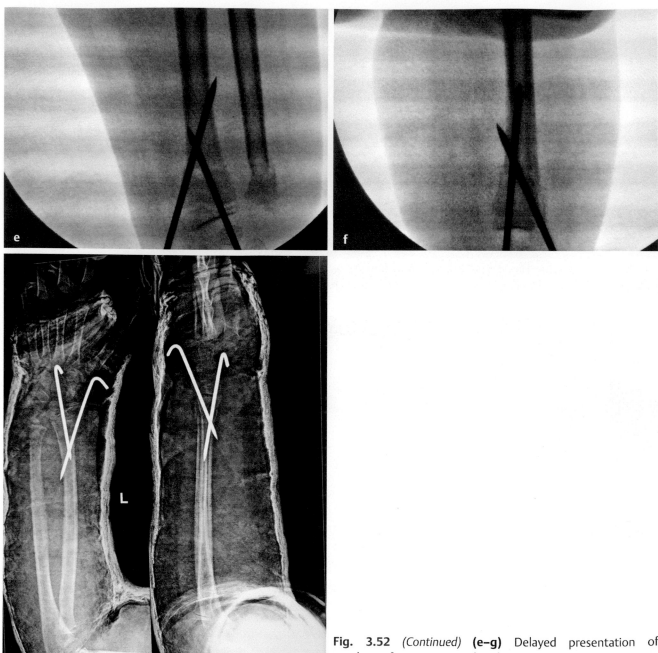

Fig. 3.52 *(Continued)* **(e–g)** Delayed presentation of quadratus fracture manipulated using percutaneous K-wire as joystick and transfixation K-wire fixation done.

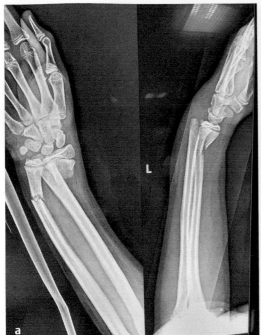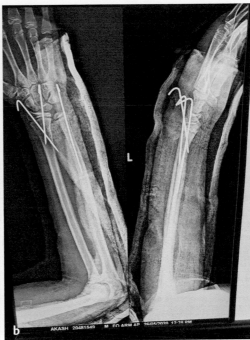

Fig. 3.53 (a, b) Volar displacement of distal radius reduced and fixed with percutaneous K-wire and ulna fracture with intramedullary K-wire.

4 Forearm

Introduction

In forearm fractures, it is important to correct both angulation and rotational deformities. The axis of rotation of the forearm bone extends from the center of the head of the radius to the insertion of the triangular fibrocartilage at the base of the styloid process of the ulna. If the relation of the forearm bones to this axis is altered by angulation, the mechanics of the radioulnar joints are deranged and permanent limitation of rotation is inevitable. Rotation deformity also limits radioulnar movement, thus affecting supination and pronation movements. Intramedullary straight K-wire and fracture transfixation cross K-wires are the two different types of K-wire fixation in forearm fractures.

K-Wire Fixation of Shaft of Radius and Ulna

Displacement of both-bone forearm fracture in children aged between 8 and 14 years can be treated by either closed manipulation, reduction, and intramedullary K-wiring or by open reduction technique and intramedullary K-wire fixation.

Closed Reduction and Intramedullary K-Wiring

In the ulna, a long K-wire of diameter 2.0 to 2.5 mm, depending on the size of the medullary canal, can be introduced in an antegrade manner from the tip of olecranon crossing the olecranon physis aiming toward the center of medullary canal in anteroposterior and lateral views under the C-arm control. Once the K-wire crosses the metaphyseal area, a cannulated plier is used to negotiate it down the medullary canal by gentle to-and-fro rotating and reciprocating movements. Once the K-wire reaches the fracture site, by traction and appropriate rotation, and by correcting the angulation, the fracture is reduced; the wire is passed across into the opposite fragment medullary canal and the tip positioned up to the metaphyseal area of the ulna head without crossing the distal physis. Wire entering from epiphysis, crossing the physis to pass into the intramedullary canal must be done with minimal attempts. Too many pricks through the epiphysis are not advisable in order to prevent growth disturbance. Passing a single wire does not cause any growth disturbance.

Radius fracture is fixed by passing a K-wire from the mid-dorsum of the distal radius in retrograde fashion. An entry point was made by a drill in an oblique fashion at metaphyseal area proximal to the distal physis. By volar flexing the wrist fully, the K-wire is introduced through the drill hole with slight bend at tip to become parallel to the shaft of the distal fragment for easy entry into the medullary canal. Sometimes the K-wire does not enter the medullary canal easily; it may go in an oblique manner hitching the volar cortex and may not proceed further. A small short bend at the tip of the K-wire may help to pass into the medullary canal by hitching the convex surface of the bend on the far cortex and tip pointing intramedullary. Always ensure this by checking the anteroposterior and lateral views for the placement of wire, their direction, and progress. By gentle rocking movement using a cannulated plier or cannulated T-clamp Jacob chuck, the wire can be advanced in, negotiating through the fracture site with the usual manipulative technique and into the proximal fragment. The wire can be positioned proximally up to the metaphyseal area of the radial neck without crossing the radial head physis. These wires are kept outside the skin. An above-elbow slab is given at the end of the procedure to control rotation for a minimum period of 6 weeks until the fracture heals and the wires are removed after radiological evidence of healing.

If the fracture radius is in distal one-fourth of shaft, it may be difficult to get a stable fixation with this type of entry. Other techniques of K-wire entry as described below are also useful for stable fixation of radius.

Radius wire can also be entered through the tip of styloid process but one need to cross the physis which is not necessary in dorsal entry. The advantage is easy entry and negotiation into the medullary canal compared to dorsal entry, which is in a more straight-line course. The first choice is metaphyseal entry rather than the epiphyseal entry and only in attempted failure through metaphysis, an epiphyseal entry is done.

Intramedullary wire passed in the distal radius from radial styloid needs prebending as it may touch the opposite cortex in an angle without entering the medullary canal. The sequence of steps in performing this technique is as follows:

1. Pass a K-wire (2.5 mm) from styloid into the medullary canal in a desired angle after predrilling.
2. The K-wire sharp tip is cut slightly prebent and negotiated through the same entry point using cannulated plier by rocking movements (**Fig. 4.1a, b**).
3. Metaphyseal fractures may require cross K-wire instaed of intramedullary K-wire.

Radius wire can also be entered easily from mid-dorsum along the line of medullary canal from dorsal articular surface by volar flexing the wrist completely. Though it is technically easy, it is theoretically damaging the articular surface and also has the disadvantage of crossing the physis. Antegrade K-wire through fracture site in open reduction also exits in the same manner for ante-retrograde wiring.

Open Reduction and Intramedullary K-Wiring

In open reduction of ulna fracture, the K-wire is introduced in a retrograde manner into the proximal fragment first, through the fracture site to exit at olecranon tip. The fracture is reduced anatomically and the wire is driven in an antegrade manner into the distal ulnar shaft to park at the distal ulnar head metaphysis. In open reduction of radius fracture, the K-wire is introduced in an antegrade manner into the distal fragment first through the fracture site to exit at wrist level dorsally, by keeping the wrist in maximum palmar flexion. The wire is then driven in a retrograde manner into the proximal

radial shaft after perfect reduction up to the proximal metaphyseal level.

Many times displaced pediatric/adolescent both-bone fractures of forearm are treated with intramedullary K-wiring of both radius and ulna fractures after closed reduction. Sometimes single-bone K-wiring is done and other bone fracture is treated with plaster of Paris (POP) cast after closed manipulation. The indications for single-bone K-wiring in both-bone fractures are as follows:

- Most displaced fractures are fixed with percutaneous K-wire and other bone may be undisplaced or greenstick fracture which can be maintained with closed reduction and above-elbow cast application.
- In displaced both-bone fracture, ulna fracture reduction is the key as this bone is nice and straight; achieving the length and correcting the angulation with straight K-wire from olecranon tip will get the radius out of length. If there is no angulation of radius even if there is complete translation, it can be treated with above-elbow POP cast in ideal forearm rotation.

Case Scenarios

Case Scenario 1

Displaced both-bone forearm fractures treated with intramedullary K-wire. The entry point for the K-wire is the dorsum of the distal end for the radius and olecranon for the ulna. (**Fig. 4.2a–f**).

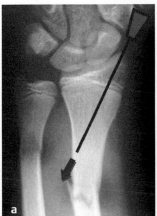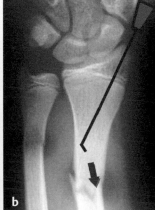

Fig. 4.1 (a, b) Sharp tip of K-wire was cut to make it blunt and then a small bend was given at the tip to negotiate the far cortex to enter intramedullary in the radius.

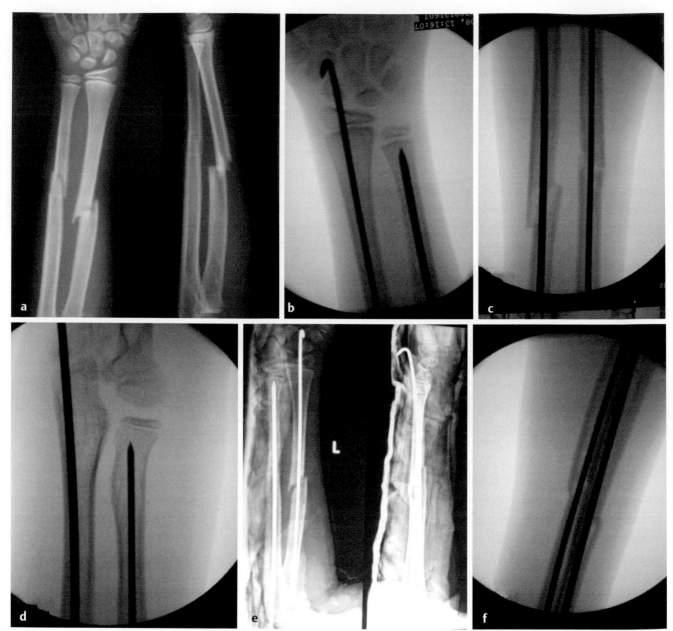

Fig. 4.2 (a–f) Displaced fracture forearm treated with intramedullary K-wire through olecranon tip for ulna fracture and through the Lister tubercle for radius fracture.

Case Scenario 2

Displaced both-bone forearm fracture and K-wiring both radius and ulna in a 13-year-old boy (**Fig. 4.3**). Closed anatomical reduction was obtained. Ulna intramedullary 3 mm K-wire was passed from the olecranon tip straight into the shaft reducing the fracture. Radius K-wire was inserted from mid-dorsum of wrist straight intramedullary through the shaft reducing the fracture spanning the whole length as shown in the picture.

Case Scenario 3

Single-bone radius forearm fracture with angulation corrected with intramedullary K-wire from the distal radius (**Fig. 4.4a, b**).

Case Scenario 4

Blunt-tip K-wire with slight prebend to negotiate into the medullary canal without abutting far cortex (**Fig. 4.5a, b**). A 9-year-old boy had proximal third

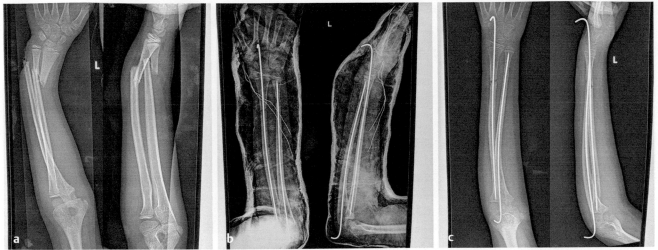

Fig. 4.3   (a–c) Closed anatomical reduction obtained. Ulna intramedullary 3-mm K-wire passed from the olecranon tip straight into the shaft reducing the fracture. Radius K-wire inserted from mid-dorsum of wrist straight intramedullary through the shaft, reducing the fracture spanning the whole length.

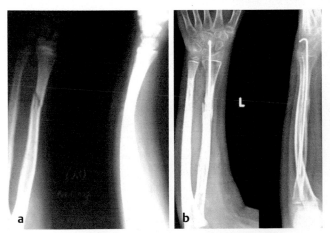

Fig. 4.4   (a, b) Displaced single-bone radius fracture of forearm treated with intramedullary K-wire.

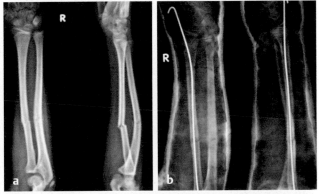

Fig. 4.5   (a, b) Displaced radius fracture was reduced with intramedullary K-wire which reduced the greenstick ulna fracture without the need for an ulnar wire and above-elbow POP cast was given.

both-bone fracture, with displacement of the radius fracture and angulation of the ulna fracture. As mentioned previously, the K-wire was passed from radial styloid after predrilling. The tip of the K-wire was prebent and negotiated through the medullary canal by gentle oscillatory movement, negotiated and passed through the fracture site, and parked just beneath the proximal radius physis. As the angulation of the ulna got corrected spontaneously, it was decided to treat with plaster. A snug-fitting above-elbow POP cast was given for 6 weeks.

Case Scenario 5

In a displaced both-bone fracture forearm, it is routine to start K-wiring of the ulna through olecranon tip being in a straight line and easy to pass. Subsequently, if the radius falls into place anatomically, this can be treated by application of an above-elbow cast as shown here and there is no need for K-wiring of the radius (**Fig. 4.6a–c**).

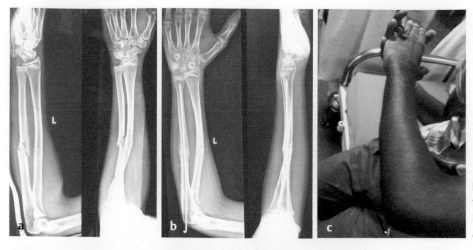

Fig. 4.6 (a–c) Both-bone forearm fracture treated with intramedullary K-wire for ulna and above elbow cast.

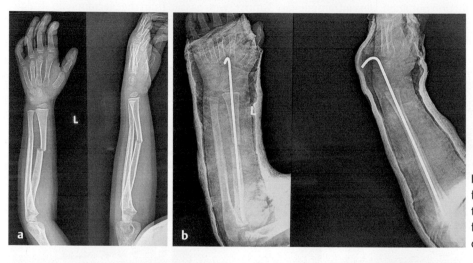

Fig. 4.7 (a, b) Both-bone forearm fracture with displaced radius treated with intramedullary K-wire fixation for radius and above elbow cast

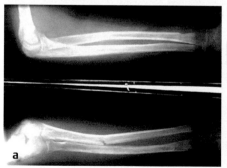
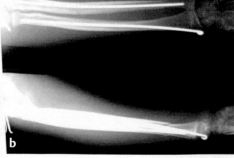

Fig. 4.8 (a, b) Intramedullary K-wire is definitely a better option in segmental fracture forearm in children.

Case Scenario 6

Displaced radius fracture with greenstick fracture of ulna (**Fig. 4.7a, b**). The angulated, displaced radius fracture was manipulated but acceptable reduction was not obtained. Hence a percutaneous straight 2.5-mm K-wire from mid-dorsum of radius was passed intramedullary through the fracture site after obtaining good reduction by closed means. The greenstick fracture of ulna was corrected and an above-elbow cast was applied. The K-wire and cast was retained for a period of 6 weeks.

Case Scenario 7

Segmental radius fracture with ulna fracture treated with intramedullary K-wire (**Fig. 4.8a, b**).

Case Scenario 8

Distal-third both-bone forearm fracture (**Fig. 4.9a–q**). Distal-third both-bone fracture of forearm in a kid can be treated by closed manipulation with or without K-wire fixation and an above-elbow cast. In an obese or a big child or when the fracture is unstable, a percutaneous K-wire fixation is mandatory. Here after closed manipulation and reduction two cross K-wires were inserted to transfix the radius fracture in good alignment because the child was obese. The fracture transfixation done with one mediolateral K-wire and the other K-wire in an anteroposterior direction. It was started from distal fragment which was a wide metaphyseal zone to the proximal shaft which is narrow thick cortex. The starting point of entry was at 1 cm distal to the fracture site and entered the near cortex at an angle of 30 degrees to the shaft of radius. After crossing the fracture site, the far cortex entry into the proximal fragment will be better felt with the resistance. A counterpressure while entering the far cortex might be necessary. Too much of axial force at this point of time may displace the fragments. It is preferable to run the drill in high speed and with less axial pressure. Once the far cortex penetration was done, the drill must be stopped abruptly without too much of overshooting of K-wire into the soft tissues. Generally backing out of K-wire because of overshooting tip will weaken the fixation and loosening can happen. As the reduction of ulna was satisfactory after fixing the radius it was left alone to be immobilized with above-elbow molded cast in the midprone position.

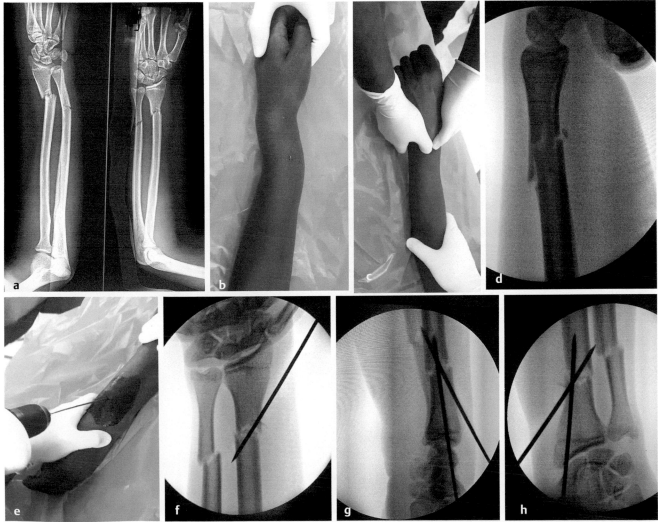

Fig. 4.9 **(a–h)** Distal third both bone fracture in a kid treated by closed manipulation and two transfixation K-wires in two planes. (*Continued*)

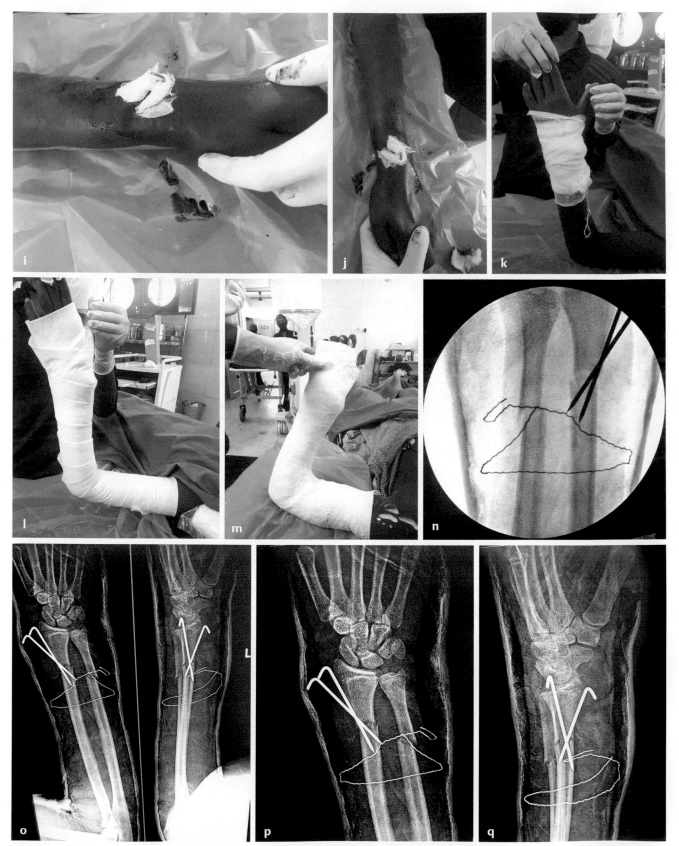

Fig. 4.9 (*Continued*) **(i–q)** Distal third both bone fracture in a kid treated by closed manipulation and two transfixation K-wires in two planes.

Case Scenario 9

Distal shaft radius and ulna fracture in a 14-year-old child (**Fig. 4.10a–e**). Most of distal forearm fractures in children above the age of 10 and below 14 years may require closed reduction and percutaneous K-wire fixation. In distal radius maintaining the traction, two cross K-wires in anteroposterior and mediolateral plane were passed from distal to proximal fragment starting 1 cm below the fracture line and entering obliquely at an angle of 30 degrees to the shaft to cross the fracture and engage on the far cortex of the proximal fragment. One must be gentle in passing the first wire as too much pressure while drilling the cortices may displace the fragments. Before entering the far cortex, both views must be done to ensure there is no angulation or displacement or marginal fixation. The second wire was passed in similar fashion in the other plane. Note the obliquity of the K-wire must not be parallel to the fracture plane and it must be perpendicular or at obtuse angle to the fracture

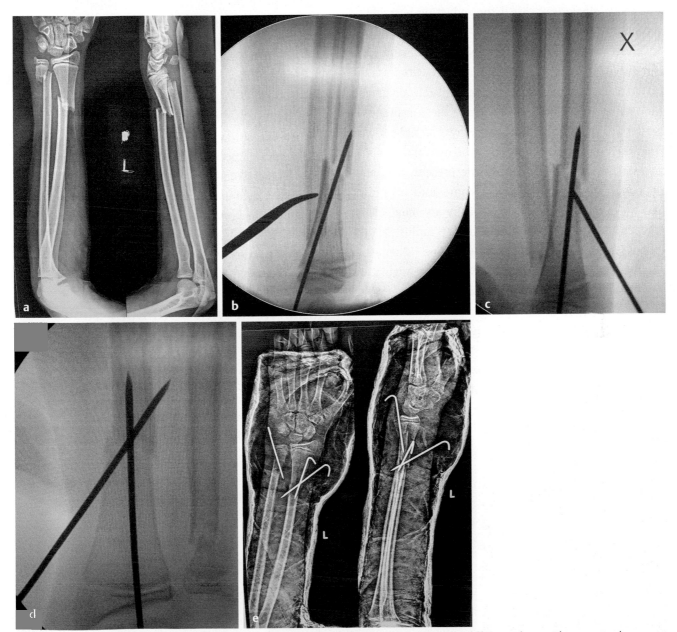

Fig. 4.10 (**a–e**) Distal radius and ulna fracture fixed with two transfixation K-wires in different planes. The wrong placement of the K-wires as shown in (**c**) may not hold the proximal fragment. Here the K-wire was parallel to fracture fragment, instead it should be perpendicular.

plane for better biomechanical fixation. An above-elbow cast is necessary for a period of 5 to 6 weeks. Wires were removed after adequate callus formation by the end of 6 weeks and mobilized further.

Case Scenario 10

Fracture midshaft radius and ulna in a 10-year-old child treated with single-bone K-wiring (**Fig. 4.11a, b**). Generally displaced angulated both-bone forearm fracture in a child can be treated by closed manipulation and above-elbow POP cast if the reduction is stable or acceptable. If not, percutaneous K-wiring would be sufficient to maintain the reduction. Normally ulna fracture is reduced and fixed with percutaneous K-wire from the tip of olecranon correcting the length and alignment. Ulna being a straight bone and along the subcutaneous border, it is easy to fix and reduce by a straight K-wire from the tip of olecranon through the olecranon epiphysis into the medullary canal. In the present case, once ulna was fixed, radius fracture came into alignment and the reduction was maintained by an above-elbow POP cast. For anterior angulation of radius, above-elbow forearm cast in pronation was done (Mnemonic: Andhra Pradesh Police Station, A-Anterior angulation, P-Pronation and P-Posterior Angulation, S-Supination).

Quadratus Fracture Forearm

Distal one-fourth both-bone fracture of the forearm in a child is common and it can be reduced by closed manipulation. Maintenance of unstable fracture or remanipulation because of loss of reduction in POP cast warrants K-wire fixation. First K-wire was passed from the dorsal cortex of distal radius 1 cm away from the fracture site in an oblique angulation of 30 to 60 degrees in order to pass through the fracture and engage the volar cortex of proximal radius. It is not passed through the epiphysis. The lateral view was checked now to ensure that there was no angulation at the fracture site. Second K-wire was passed from the lateral cortex of distal radius 1 cm distal to the fracture site in an oblique angulation and advanced through the fracture and to the medial cortex of proximal fragment. Again, the position was checked in both anteroposterior and lateral views in image intensifier. Once two cross K-wires were applied in two different planes to secure the radius fracture in anatomical position, an above-elbow POP cast was applied in midprone position and ulna fracture was kept in a reasonable position of reduction without additional fixation (**Fig. 4.12a–d**).

Another example of distal-fourth radius and ulna fracture treated with cross K-wiring of radius fracture after closed manipulation and reduction (**Fig. 4.13a, b**). The ulna fracture was taken care by above-elbow cast immobilization.

Radial Neck with Both-Bone Shaft Fracture

Open reduction and internal fixation with plate and screws were done for the radius and ulna shaft fractures

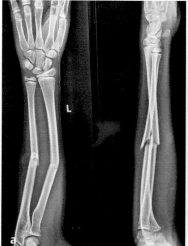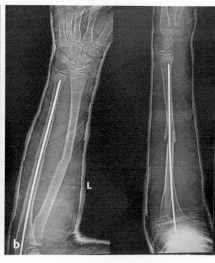

Fig. 4.11 (a, b) Displaced angulated both-bone fragment in a child treated with single intramedullary K-wire for ulna fracture and above elbow cast applied to hold the reduction of radius fracture.

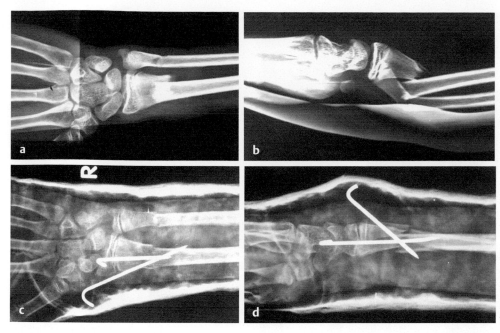

Fig. 4.12 (a–d) Displaced distal-fourth forearm fracture reduced and fixed with two metaphyseal cross K-wires in two dimensions.

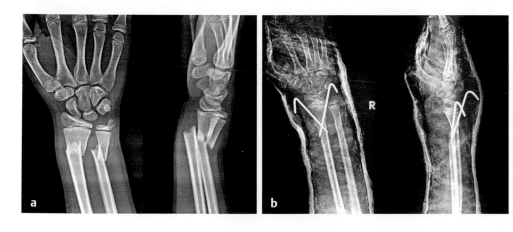

Fig. 4.13 (a, b) Displaced quadratus fracture treated with closed manipulation reduction and percutaneous cross K-wiring.

of the forearm. The radial neck fracture was transfixed with a percutaneous K-wire from lateral aspect of the head through the safe zone by a transfixation K-wire and immobilized further with above-elbow POP splint, as shown in **Fig. 4.14a–g**.

Marginal Fracture Radial Head

Displaced marginal fracture radial head can be reduced by closed means using K-wire as a joystick to manipulate. Percutaneous K-wire was passed through the safe zone, that is, 90-degree horizontal position in supination and 90-degree vertical position in pronation. The fracture is reduced and transfixed as shown in **Fig. 4.15a–e**.

Monteggia Fracture Dislocation

As shown in **Fig. 4.16a–c**, a small child with Monteggia fracture dislocation with anterior displacement and angulation was treated by percutaneous K-wire passed from the tip of the olecranon intramedullary into the ulna shaft fracture. Fracture was reduced and fixed by intramedullary K-wire spanning the ulnar length out. This automatically reduced the radial head dislocation. An above-elbow POP slab in supination was given to maintain the reduction for a period of 4 weeks until adequate callus was formed.

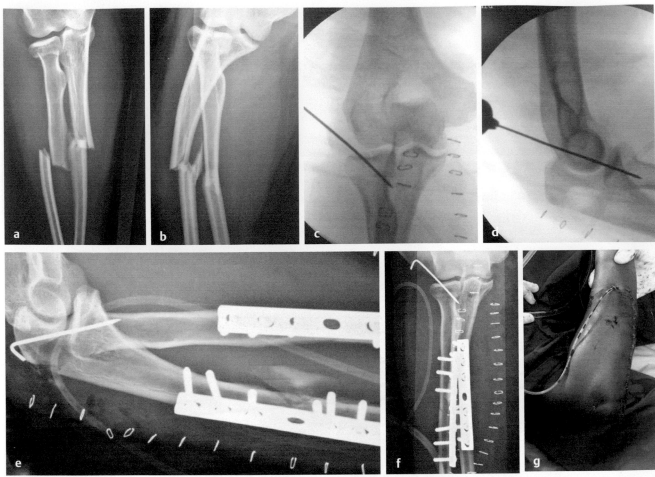

Fig. 4.14 (a–g) Radial neck with radius and ulna diaphyseal fracture treated with plating of shaft fracture, and radial neck secured with percutaneous K-wire through safe zone from head to shaft and the clinical picture showing the entry.

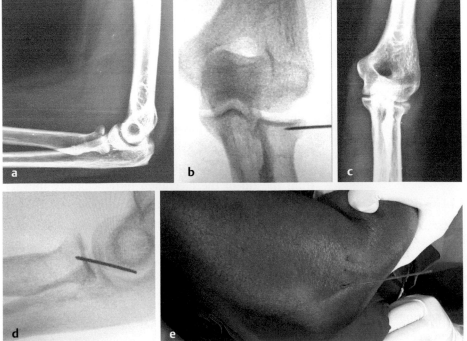

Fig. 4.15 (a–e) Marginal fracture radial head fixed with subchondral K-wire through safe zone.

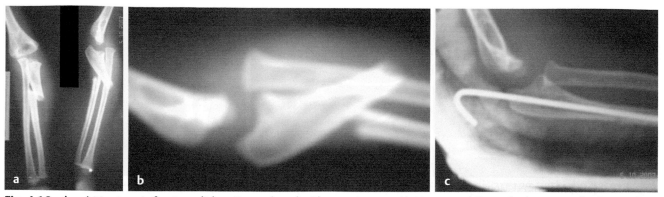

Fig. 4.16 **(a–c)** Monteggia fracture dislocation reduced with percutaneous K-wire passed through olecranon physis to reduce the ulna fracture. Once the ulna fracture was reduced and out of length, radial head dislocation was reduced automatically.

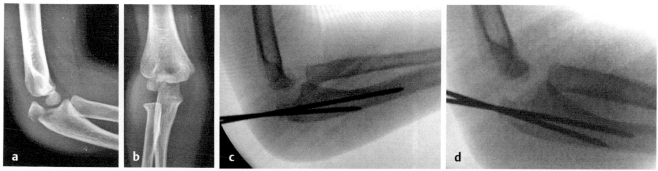

Fig. 4.17 **(a–d)** Intra-articular fracture olecranon treated with two olecranon transfixation K-wires.

Monteggia Variant Fracture

As shown in **Fig. 4.17a–d**, a child with displaced proximal ulna fracture with radial neck fracture was treated with closed percutaneous K-wire fixation because of associated blistering of skin and swelling. The ulna fracture was reduced anatomically with no step in the joint and two K-wires were used here as one was directly entering the medullary canal without much hold and the other wire purchase was good in both cortices. This also helps in rotational stability.

Old Monteggia Fracture Dislocation

Anterior dislocation of radial head with malunited ulna with anterior angulation was treated by corrective osteotomy of the ulna at previous fracture site, reduction of radial head dislocation, and fixation of the ulna in the desired degree of posterior angulation in order to maintain radial head articulation with capitellum. After fixation of the ulna with plate, the radial head was

subluxing; hence, a radiocapitellar K-wire was passed to maintain the reduction for a period of 4 weeks, as shown in **Fig. 4.18a–c**. Above-elbow POP slab was applied and the K-wire was removed after 4 weeks.

Distal Radius and Ulna Fracture with Supracondylar Fracture of Ipsilateral Arm

A 14-year-old boy sustained roller machine injury with distal radius and distal ulna metaphyseal fracture, and supracondylar humerus comminuted fracture. Supracondylar fracture was fixed first after closed manipulation and reduction of the fracture with two medial and two lateral K-wires as shown in **Fig. 4.19a–e**.

The distal radius quadratus fracture was reduced anatomically and maintained with two K-wires, one passed from the dorsal cortex of distal fragment about 1 cm away from the fracture with 60-degrees angulation, so that it crossed the fracture and engaged the proximal fragment 1 cm away. Fixation in another plane was done

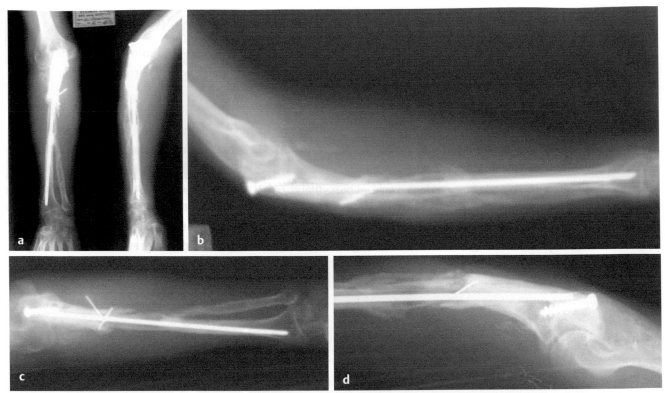

Fig. 4.21 **(a–d)** Extensive bone and soft tissue loss in the forearm treated with fusion of the ulna to radius by a square intramedullary nail and bone grafting at cross union site with transfixation K-wire for rotational stability.

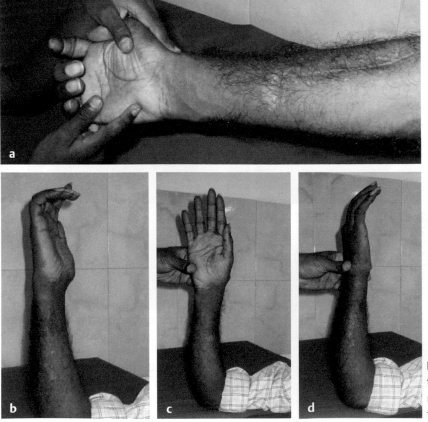

Fig. 4.22 **(a–d)** Clinical outcome showing the relative supination/pronation movement preservation and presently, he is a truck driver by occupation.

5 Elbow

Supracondylar Fracture

Supracondylar fracture humerus is most common in children between 5 and 8 years of age due to a fall on an outstretched hand. Treatment is usually closed reduction and percutaneous pinning. Most common is the extension type (95%), and rarest is flexion type (5%). In closed reduction of extension type with posteromedial displacement, forearm is pronated and hyperflexed. In extension type with posterolateral displacement, forearm is supinated and hyperflexed. With patient in supine position on a radiolucent table, for a right supracondylar fracture, holding the forearm in his/her right hand and both the condyles between the index finger and the thumb of the left hand, the surgeon can feel the position of the distal fragment. In this position, gentle traction is given with the forearm in extension and supination. The assistant should give countertraction by holding the upper arm and stabilizing the proximal fragment by applying pressure on the anterior aspect of proximal humerus. Once the mediolateral tilt and rotation are aligned to the proximal humerus, gentle flexion of the forearm is done with the surgeon's thumb over the olecranon to correct the posterior angulation. In a well-built patient, sometimes it is necessary to use both the thumbs to give a good push. Full flexion is only possible when the fragments align in proper position. Normally, full pronation is necessary to correct the lateral opening. it is necessary to keep the forearm in supination to achieve good reduction in posterolateral displacement. Clinically, the point of elbow should be in line with the shaft of humerus. Holding the forearm in maximum flexion, reduction is checked under image control in both anteroposterior (AP) (shoot through) and lateral views. When taking a lateral view, one should not rotate the forearm as a lever; rather the upper arm is rotated holding the reduction steadily. Or, the C-arm itself can be rotated to take a true lateral in supine 90-degree abducted arm. At this point, if the reduction is stable, an above-elbow slab is applied in flexion (**Fig. 5.1a–e**).

If the fracture is unstable, percutaneous K-wire fixation is done. In reduced position, two K-wires of 1.6/2 mm diameter are passed in a crisscross manner, from lateral and medial condyle or two K-wires from lateral condyle in divergent fashion engaging the opposite cortex. A folded sheet is kept under the upper arm and the assistant should hold it flexed fully in the reduced position. This approximately gives a 30-degree angle up to the humerus with respect to the flat arm table. The K-wire is entered keeping in line with the humerus, which is 30 degrees up from the arm table, a position of ease for surgeon to work (**Fig. 5.2**).

Cross K-wiring for Supracondylar Humerus Fracture

For cross-wire fixation, the first wire is passed from lateral side, and because the center of the capitellum is in line with anterior aspect of humeral shaft, the pin must be directed slightly posteriorly. The wire is inserted through the capitellum, and then through the distal humeral physis. In general, the pin is aimed at 30 to 60 degree angle to the arm sideways and 10 degrees posteriorly directed; one should avoid the olecranon fossa and should come to rest along the far cortex approximately 3 cm above the fracture line. Insert a lateral pin first to obtain stability as shown in **Fig. 5.3a–g** and **Video 5.1**.

The medial pin is passed obliquely through the medial epicondyle and just proximal to olecranon fossa. One needs to protect the ulnar nerve. It is to be noted that with flexion, the ulnar nerve can subluxate over the medial epicondyle placing it at risk with a medial pin insertion. Because of ulnar nerve subluxation, some

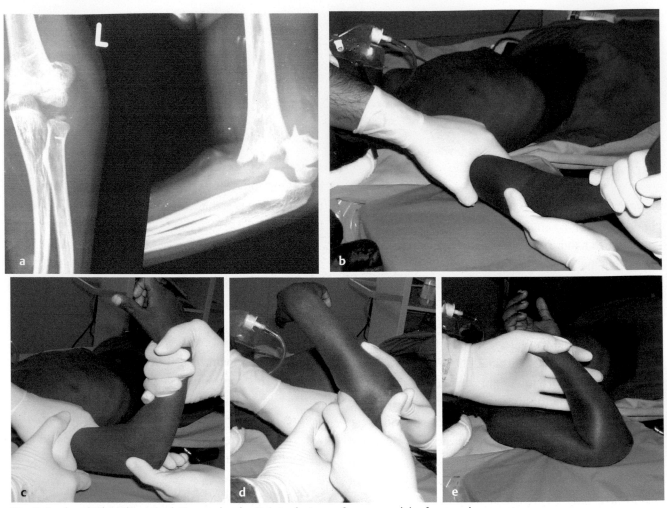

Fig. 5.1 (a–e) Closed manipulation and reduction technique of supracondylar fracture humerus.

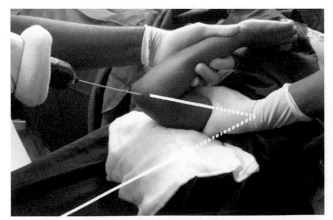

Fig. 5.2 In supine position with folded sheet under the elbow, K-wire can be easily passed through the condyle directing toward the humeral shaft.

surgeons always place the lateral pin first (with elbow hyperflexed), which gives stability. Once the lateral pin has been inserted, the surgeon can then bring the elbow out to less flexion, 60- to 80-degree flexion (decreasing ulnar nerve subluxation), before the placement of the medial pin. The surgeon's thumb can milk the ulnar nerve back into its posterior position and hold it there. If an excessive soft tissue swelling is present, consider making a small incision through the skin over the medial epicondyle and then spreading with hemostat, and use K-wire drill sleeve to further protect the ulnar nerve. When medial K-wire is inserted, look for any twitch over the little finger as K-wire on the nerve will cause irritation and twitch. Because medial epicondyle is slightly

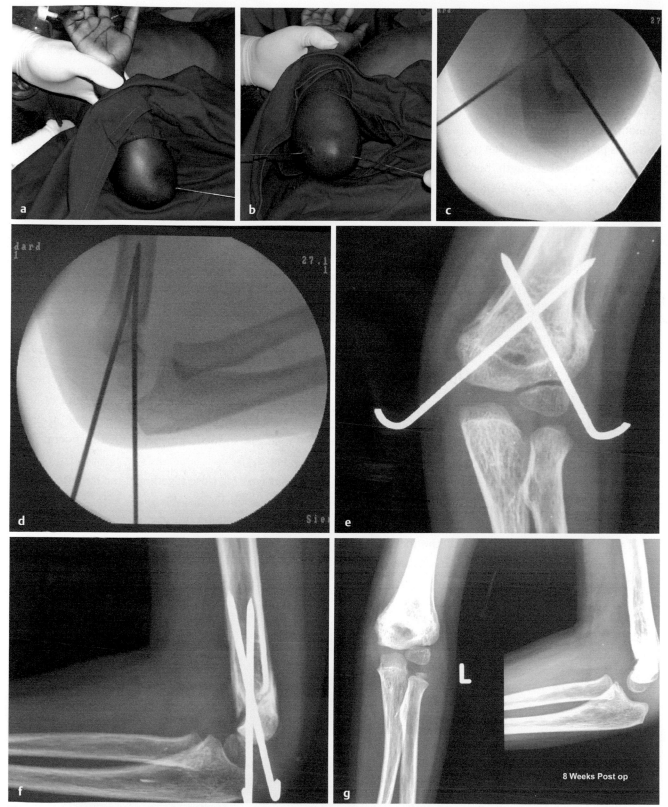

Fig. 5.3 **(a–g)** Lateral K-wire is passed first and then the medial K-wire in a crisscross fashion.

posterior to the shaft, direct the medial pin slightly anterior and also ensure that the medial pin enters straight into the epicondyle rather than distal to the epicondyle. The medial wire will often appear more transverse than the lateral pin. The pin should cross each other 1.5 to 2 cm above the fracture line.

Biomechanical studies of stability have proven that two cross pins are stronger than two lateral pins on evaluating the torsional strength. But two divergent lateral pins are better than two parallel or convergent lateral pins. Again three divergent construct lateral pins are equivalent to cross pins in stiffness, except in valgus.

Clinical results presently favor two lateral divergent K-wires because of comparable construct stiffness in order to avoid injury to ulnar nerve (4%) except in special occasions. Cross pinning is also a good option, if one follows the steps to avoid ulnar nerve injury by meticulous technique.

Lateral Entry K-Wire Fixation for Supracondylar Fracture

A 1.5 mm K-wire is inserted from lateral condyle after closed reduction. This can be of two types:

1. Two parallel lateral pins.
2. Two divergent lateral pins.

Most lateral wire is passed from the lateral condyle, lateral to the olecranon fossa, into the lateral column at the fracture site and proximally into the metaphyseal shaft of distal humerus medial cortex. Because divergent K-wires are preferable for better rotational torque control, next wire is passed from the lateral condyle entering the medial column crossing the fracture site and into the medial metaphyseal cortex. The pins that cross at the fracture line close to each other are rotationally unstable and must be avoided. The major advantage is that damage to ulnar nerve from medial entry K-wire is avoided. If the fracture exits very distally on the lateral side then it is difficult to stabilize with lateral pins alone and a medial entry K-wire is necessary.

Sometimes third K-wire is necessary if the reduction is rotationally unstable even after two pins. Here, there are two options, namely, all three lateral pins, with the third pin through the middle column (olecranon fossa), or two lateral and one medial pin.

Causes for Loss of Reduction

- Inadequate reduction.
- Inadequate fixation where the pin has missed the fixation of near cortex or the far cortex or intramedullary position of tip of K-wire or short purchase (not engaging sufficient bone in proximal and distal fragment) from the fracture site (**Fig. 5.4**).
- Pins crossing close together at the fracture site will be rotationally unstable.
- Severe comminution at the fracture site with unstable reduction warranting additional third K-wire.
- Thin K-wires.

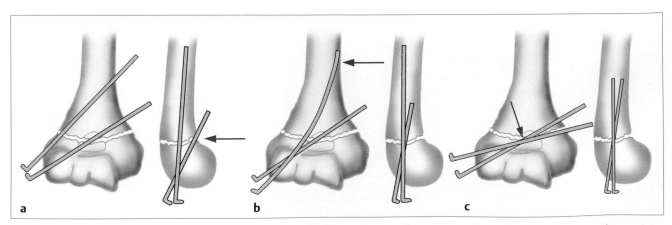

Fig. 5.4 Pitfalls in pin fixation. **(a)** Anterior pin failing to fix the proximal bone. **(b)** Demonstrates unicortical purchase of the pin which is undesirable. **(c)** Depicts pins crossing the fracture site are too close giving little mechanical stability.

Case Scenario 1

Lateral K-wiring for supracondylar humerus fracture: In lateral entry two K-wire techniques, two divergent K-wires are passed with short and long oblique purchase from the capitellum to the medial cortex of the proximal humerus, as shown in **Fig. 5.5a–c**. The long purchase oblique K-wire should not be too proud as it may impale on brachial artery or ulnar nerve, causing iatrogenic injury. Always check for the stability and feel the distal pulse at the end of the procedure. An above-elbow slab in 90-degree flexion is given in midprone position, leaving the wrist and hand free for movements. Check X-ray is taken at the end of 3 to 4 weeks, and if sufficient callus is seen, the wires are removed and active-elbow range of movements is started.

Case Scenario 2

Inadequate reduction leading to wrong placement of K-wires. **Fig. 5.6a, b** shows how wrongly sometimes a K-wire can miss the distal fragment. This is a common mistake in supracondylar fracture humerus. In this case, the medial K-wire has missed the distal fragment and entered directly through the fracture into the proximal fragment humerus supracondylar area, and lateral fragment K-wire has entered the capitellum, exited the bone, and again gone into the proximal fragment of humerus. This problem is caused by inadequate reduction and is bound to fail. For assessing the true lateral, it is easy to spin the C-arm scan 90 degrees rather than rotating the elbow, which may cause loss of reduction or opening on one side causing varus/valgus tilt. One should feel the proprioception of drilling the bone both distally and proximally, and also check, if in doubt, in different positions under C-arm image guidance to prevent this technical fault.

Case Scenario 3

Distal third fracture shaft of humerus: **Fig. 5.7a–d** depicts a high supracondylar fracture, in which a long oblique K-wire from the medial and lateral condyle is passed to secure the fracture in good position as shown. Here lateral K-wiring alone may not be possible and bicolumn K-wire fixation gives the maximum stability.

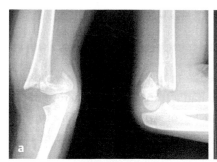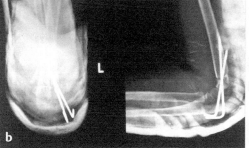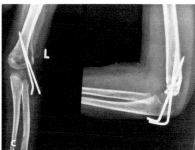

Fig. 5.5 **(a–c)** Supracondylar fractured humerus fixed with two lateral K-wires.

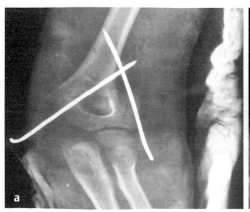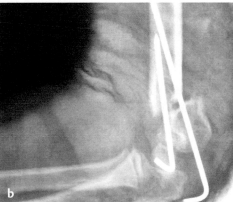

Fig. 5.6 **(a, b)** K-wire missing the proximal/distal fragment because of improper inadequate reduction.

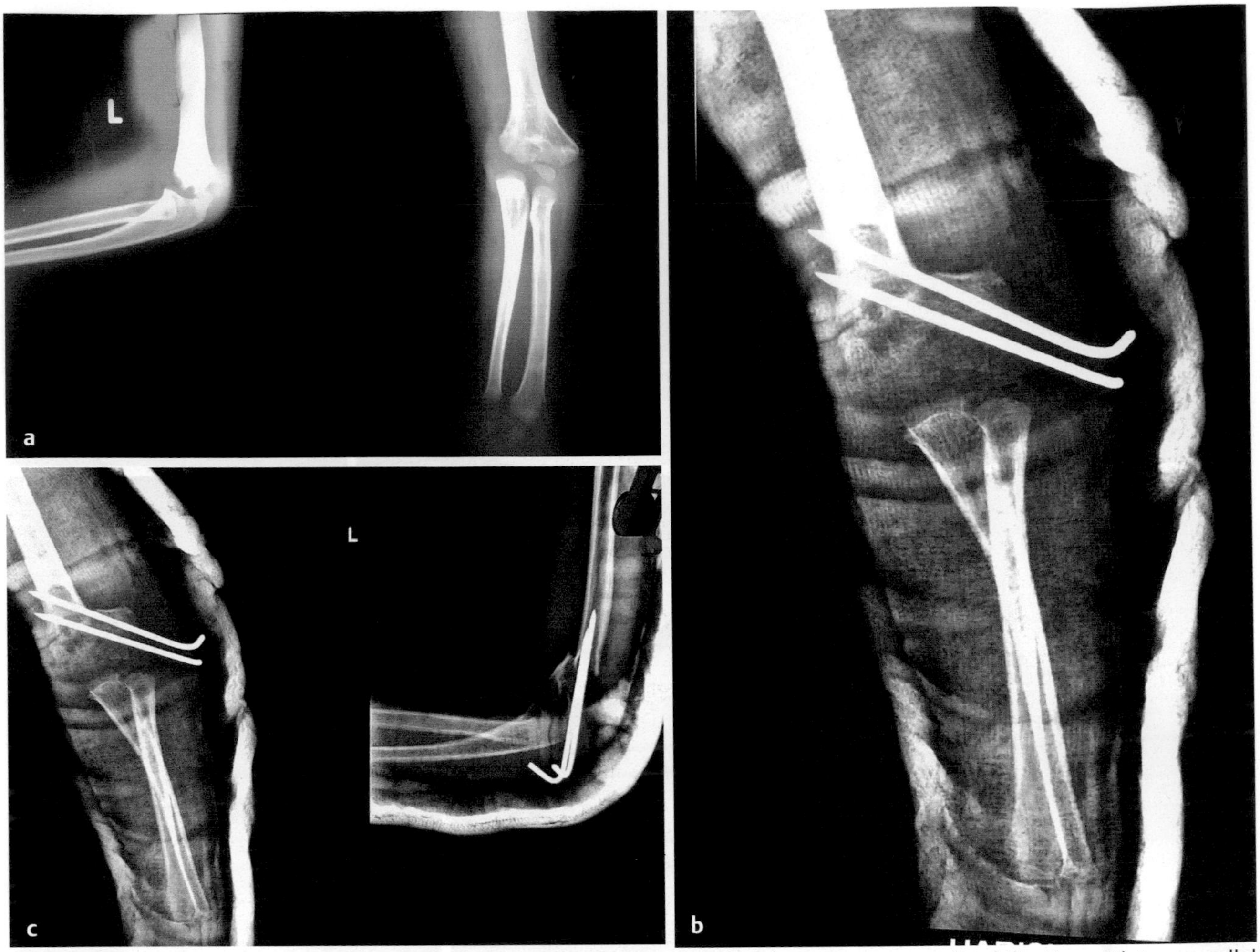

Fig. 5.10 (a–c) Cubitus varus deformity is corrected by laterally closing wedge osteotomy and stabilization with two parallel lateral K-wires.

Extension-Type Transcondylar Fracture in Elderly

Similar to children, extension-type transcondylar fractures in elderly can be well managed by transcondylar cross K-wire fixation. It is advisable to insert three or four K-wires from medial and lateral condyle as they become loose over a period of time because of osteoporosis in elderly. In this case, two lateral and one medial K-wires are used after anatomical reduction. For the first 6 weeks, an above-elbow POP slab is given and supervised physiotherapy in the form of active-elbow range of movement exercises is done after removing and reapplying the plaster slab every day. After 6 weeks only arm pouch and dressing at local site is done, and the patient is encouraged to do active-elbow range of movement

exercises. These wires are removed at the end of 8 weeks after confirming the radiological evidence of healing (**Fig. 5.12a–d**).

Lateral Condyle Fracture

Acute Displaced and Rotated Lateral Condyle Fracture Humerus

Displaced and rotated lateral condyle fracture by the pull of common extensor origin is an absolute indication for surgery. It should be anatomically reduced matching the articular surface by open reduction and internal fixation. Utmost care to preserve the soft tissue attachment for blood supply to the fragment is important. Smooth 2-mm K-wires are used to transfix the lateral condyle fragment.

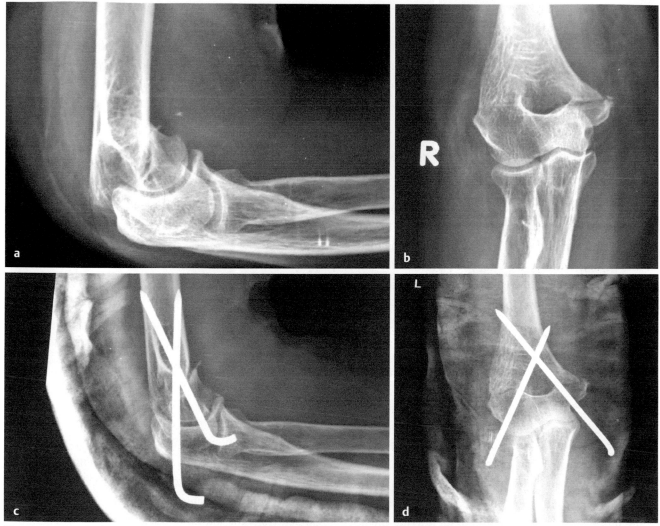

Fig. 5.11 **(a–d)** Flexion-type supracondylar fracture reduced in extension and fixed with two cross K-wires.

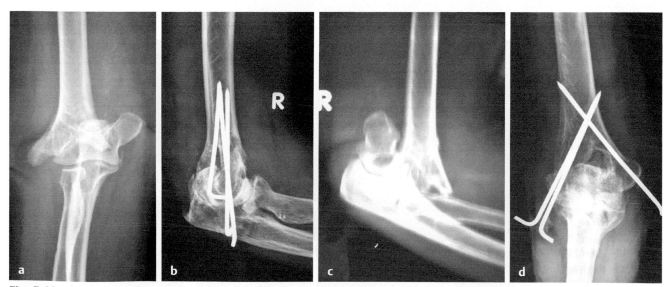

Fig. 5.12 **(a–d)** Extension-type supracondylar fracture reduced and fixed with three K-wires because of osteoporosis.

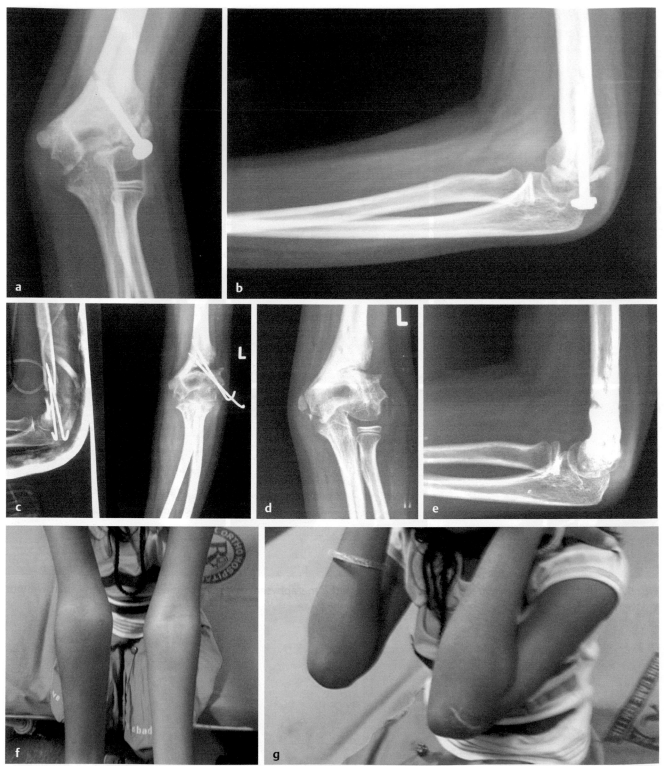

Fig. 5.16 (a–g) Malunited lateral condyle fracture with valgus deformity (previous open reduction and screw fixation) treated with lateral opening wedge osteotomy and fixation with two lateral K-wires.

Bicondylar Fracture Humerus

Case Scenario 1

"T" intercondylar fracture humerus is a rare fracture in children (**Fig. 5.17a, b**). A 14-year-old boy fell down and landed on his elbow when he was riding a horse. The X-ray shows anteriorly displaced condyles with personality of fracture not clear. In this situation, either we can consider a computed tomography (CT) scan or examination under anesthesia with C-arm image intensifier to get more information. The latter was performed to confirm the findings. By medial and lateral approach, the fractures were reduced and fixed with medial and lateral column K-wires in good position. Two wires on either side were used as the boy was obese and big built.

An additional above-elbow POP slab was used to support the elbow.

Case Scenario 2

This is a case of "T" intercondylar fracture of the distal humerus in a child (**Fig. 5.18a–c**). Here CT scan confirmed the extension-type supracondylar fracture with intercondylar element. As the intercondylar fracture was not much displaced, two cross K-wires were used to fix the condylar fragment from medial and lateral epicondyle. Through a miniopen medial approach a mediolateral intercondylar lag screw was applied without disturbing the ulnar nerve. An above-elbow slab is given for a period of 3 weeks and K-wires were removed at the end of 3 weeks to mobilize the elbow.

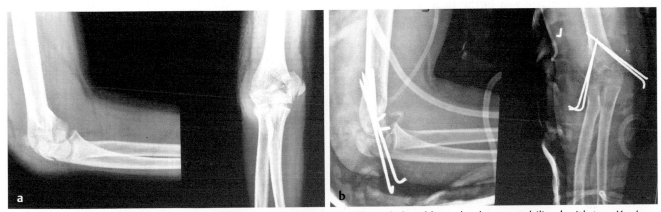

Fig. 5.17 (a, b) Intra-articular T-shaped fracture reduced and both medial and lateral columns stabilized with two K-wires on either sides.

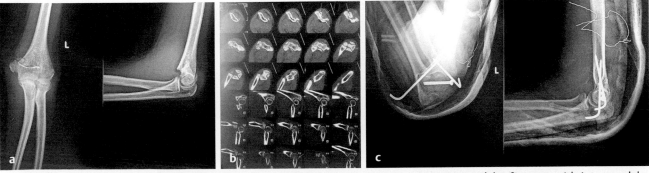

Fig. 5.18 (a–c) Computed tomography (CT) scan confirmed the extension-type supracondylar fracture with intercondylar element.

Olecranon Fracture

Olecranon Tension Band Wiring

It is a dynamic tension band wiring for the fracture. According to the tension band principle, the figure-of-eight wire is applied in the tension side of the fracture to convert the tension force into a compression force.

Patient is positioned either in lateral position with arm support or in supine position with forearm across the chest. With tourniquet control, a midline posterior skin incision is made centering the elbow joint, and fracture is exposed, reduced, and held with a hook or clamp. Then two 1.6 mm K-wires are introduced parallel to each other and they should penetrate the anteriorcortex distal to coronoid. Once the pin pierces the far cortex, it is backed out by 5 mm so that when we bend and impact the K-wire later, it will rest in the final desirable position rather than too much proud. K-wires inserted into the medullary canal without far cortex fixation are liable to back out with active-elbow movements necessitating another surgery. A 1.5 mm stainless steel wire is passed through a 2.5 mm drill hole made transversely in the ulnar shaft about 6 cm from the tip of the olecranon. Figure-of-eight tension band wiring is done by passing the stainless steel wire close to the insertion of the triceps muscle at the olecranon using cannulated hypodermic needle to pass the stainless steel wire. Once the stainless steel wire is tensioned by twisting, the knot is cut leaving 1 cm so that it can be bent over the bone

and punched to avoid any local irritation. It is preferable to have the knot on the lateral aspect of figure-of-eight rather than medial aspect as this may irritate the patient while resting the elbow on a table. Then the proximal portion of the wire is bent and buried.

Case Scenario 1

An example of the Olecranon fracture treated with tension band wiring (**Fig. 5.19a, b**)

Case Scenario 2

This is a upper ulna shaft with olecranon fracture (**Fig. 5.20a–d**). Severely osteoporotic elderly woman with upper shaft ulna fracture had plate fixation and augmentation with tension band wiring with two long intramedullary K-wires and figure-of-eight tension band stainless steel wire. The proximal screws through the plate are not having secure fixation and cannot obtain six cortices purchase, which warrants this additional fixation. A cerclage wire is also added

Case Scenario 3

In reconstructive elbow surgery olecranon osteotomy approach is better for good visualization in acute, malunited, or nonunion of distal intra-articular humerus fractures. After the fracture humerus is fixed, the olecranon is fixed back by tension band principle using two transfixing K-wires and figure-of-eight stainless steel wire, as shown in **Fig. 5.21a, b**.

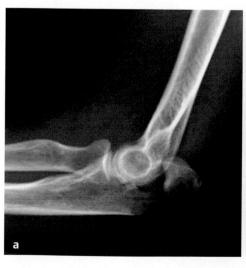
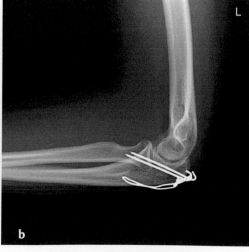

Fig. 5.19 (a, b) Olecranon fracture treated with tension band wiring.

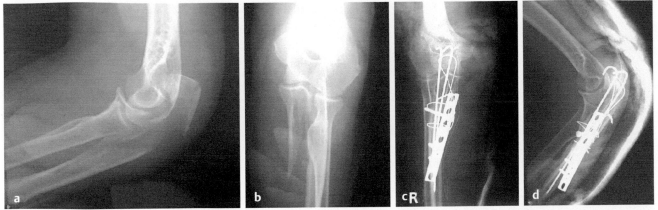

Fig. 5.20 (a–d) Upper ulna with shaft fracture stabilized with intramedullary K-wire and tension band wiring in addition to plate screw fixation.

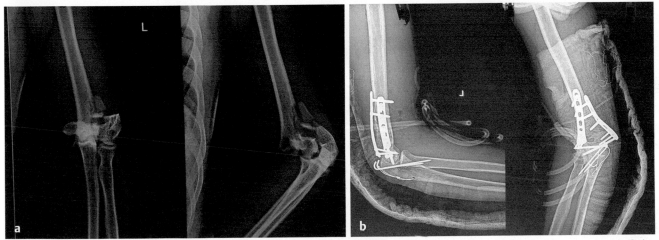

Fig. 5.21 (a, b) In intra-articular distal humerus fracture, olecranon osteotomy approach is used for reconstruction and the olecranon reattached by tension band technique.

Elbow Dislocation

Chronic Unreduced Elbow Dislocation

Case Scenario 1

Fig. 5.22a–d shows a 2-month-old injury to the elbow, which was treated by a local quack and was left unattended. Oil massage and local application triggered massive heterotopic ossification, as shown in the X-ray. Open reduction, excision of myositis ossificans in the front and back of the elbow is done by medial and lateral approach. After reduction the joint is found unstable. Hence, a 3 mm K-wire is used to transfix the humeroulnar joint starting from the middle of olecranon centering in the lateral view and directly aiming for the shaft or engaging the posterior cortex of the humeral shaft. The congruency of reduction of humeroulnar joint is checked by shoot through AP radiograph view showing "inverted V-shaped" congruity of the humeroulnar joint and lateral view of uniform congruency of the humeroulnar joint and radial head articulation centered on the capitellum.

Case Scenario 2

Unstable elbow dislocation. After closed or open reduction of elbow dislocation, if the reduction is unstable, percutaneous stabilization of humeroulnar joint may be necessary. A 3 mm K-wire is passed from the dorsal ridge of the ulna 2 cm distal to olecranon tip, keeping the elbow at 90-degree angle aiming in the lateral view of C-arm scan toward the center of the humeral shaft.

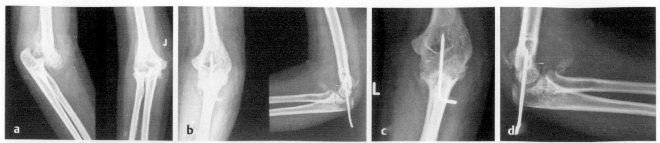

Fig. 5.22 (a–d) Open reduction of chronic unreduced dislocation of the elbow with myositis ossificans needed a transolecranon K-wire into the humeral shaft and immobilization for 4 weeks.

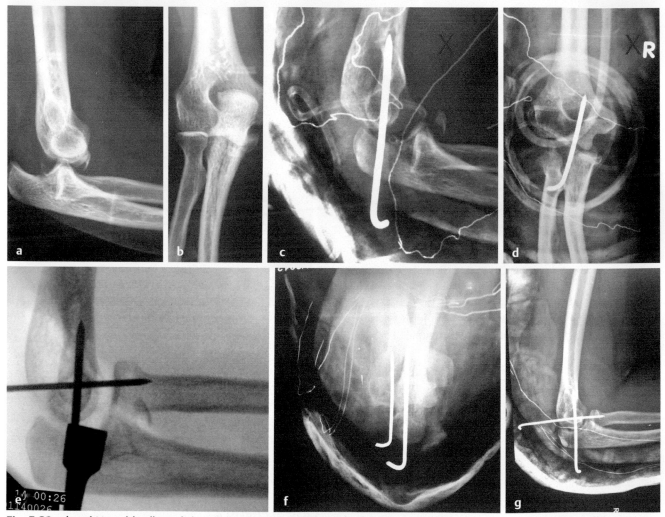

Fig. 5.23 (a–g) Unstable elbow dislocation reduced and secured with transolecranon K-wire, but the reduction is incongruent. **(c, d)** *X mark* signifies necessitated readjustment of transolecranon K-wire and additional capitelloradial K-wire.

An engagement of 2 cm crossing the joint is enough. Radiocapitellar joint alignment is checked for congruity by drawing a line along midaxis of radial shaft, which should pass through the center of capitellum. If not, the radiocapitellar joint is unreduced. A stabilization K-wire of 2.5 mm can be introduced from capitellum into the center of the radial head transfixing the joint. As shown in **Fig. 5.23a–g** slight incongruity should be critically analyzed opening of joint space and posterior dislocation of the radial head and ulnar subluxation in shoot through AP view. This could not be accepted and the procedure was redone showing the corrected congruous reduction.

Terrible Triad of Elbow

Radial head fracture with coronoid fracture and elbow dislocation is an unstable condition described by Hotchkiss. Repair and reconstruction of all the fractures will yield good results. Removal of radial head due to dislocation, comminution, or late presentation can lead on to unstable elbow. Hence, scrupulous follow-up with above-elbow POP in flexion more than 90 degrees may be necessary. If still unstable, 3 mm K wire may be used to transfix the ulnohumeral joint in congruent reduction at 90 to 100 degrees flexion and immobilization with above-elbow POP cast to prevent breakage of K-wire.

The wire must be passed from the crest of olecranon on the extensor aspect. The starting point being in line with anterior humeral line in the lateral view directing posteriorly and laterally so that the fixation is in the middle of the distal end of the humerus. Far cortex penetration at posterior distal humerus can be done if the fixation is not rigid or in an osteoporotic bone.

Case scenario 1

Coronoid fracture with marginal radial head fracture with dislocation reduced and fixed with olecrano-humerus K-wiring (**Fig. 5.24a–e**)

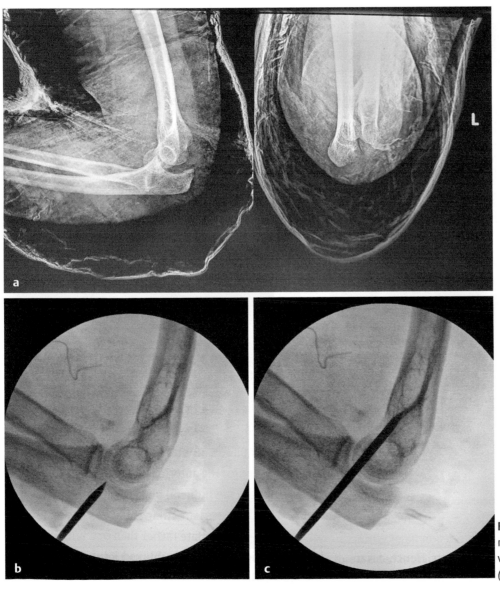

Fig. 5.24 (a–c) Unstable terrible traid of elbow stabilized with 3 mm ulnohumeral K-wire. *(Continued)*

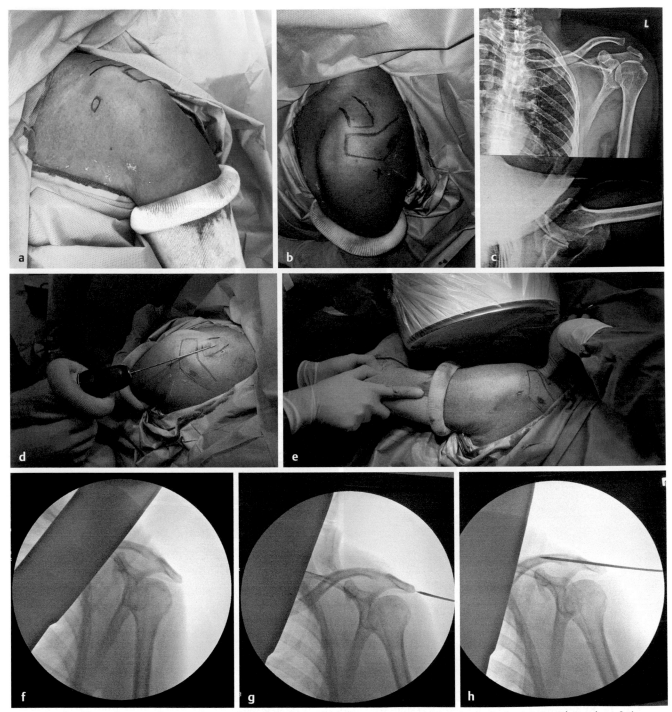

Fig. 7.3 (a–h) Surface marking with trajectory for placement of K-wire across acromioclavicular joint with implant failure.

inserted for a snug-fit intramedullary containment (**Fig. 7.4a, b**). These wires can penetrate the cortex of the medial fragment clavicle for a better purchase, but not too prominent outside the bone. Axial view is mandatory to assess the direction of the wire as shown in **Fig. 7.5a–e**.

Pull–push of the shoulder in the direction above and below was done by axially loading the humerus to demonstrate the adequate stability of fixation in AP view under a C-arm scan.

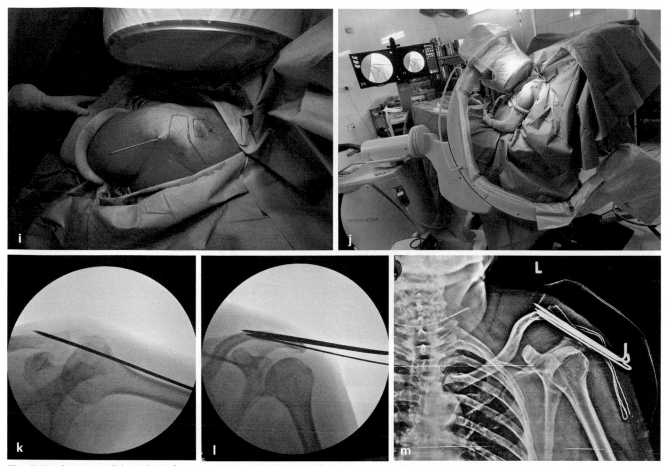

Fig. 7.3 *(Continued)* **(i–m)** Surface marking with trajectory for placement of K-wire across acromioclavicular joint with implant failure.

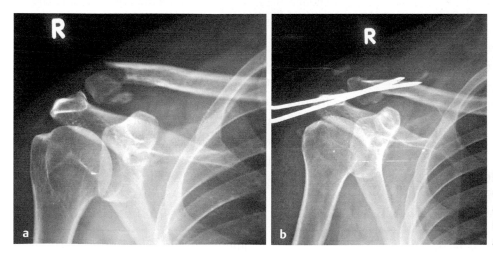

Fig. 7.4 (a, b) Lateral-end clavicle fracture fixed with transacromion acromioclavicular joint (ACJ) transfixing K-wire similar to ACJ stabilization.

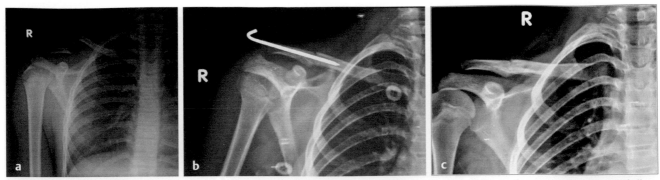

Fig. 7.8 (a–c) Displaced clavicle fracture in a child with skin tethering had open reduction and retrograde intramedullary K-wire fixation.

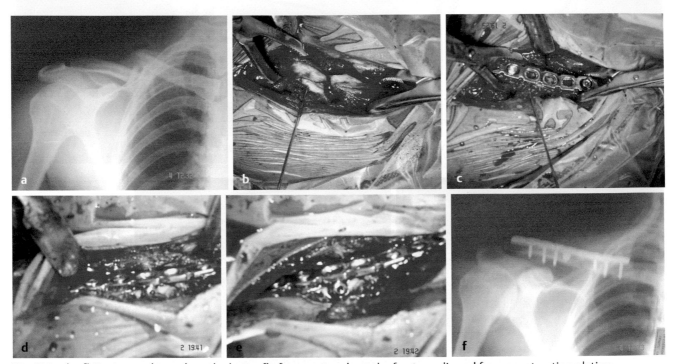

Fig. 7.9 (a–f) K-wire used to reduce the butterfly fragment and get the fracture aligned for reconstruction plating.

Clavicle Fracture Plating

Using a reconstruction locking plate for a comminuted clavicle fracture is a surgical exercise. Often, there is wedge comminution or segmental comminution that needs to match to the primary fragment like a jigsaw puzzle. These fragments were held in place by temporary fixation using thin smooth K-wire, as shown in **Fig. 7.9a–f**, before definitive fixation with the plate. Once the fragments were securely fixed with locking reconstruction plate and lag screws, the K-wire was removed.

Bilateral Shoulder Dislocation in an Epilepsy Patient (Fig. 7.10a–c)

Unstable reduction after closed manipulation of bilateral shoulder dislocation in a known epileptic patient is always a challenge. There is a high chance of recurrence of fits and redislocation. Moreover the patient had greater tuberosity fracture on the left. Both the shoulders were unstable under anesthesia and examination warranted glenohumeral fixation with a 3.5-mm thick K-wire. It is ideally started at the most lateral aspect

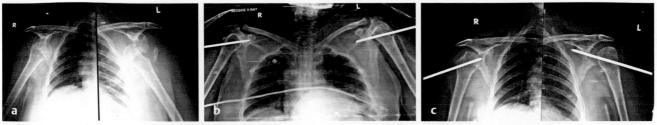

Fig. 7.10 **(a–c)** Unstable bilateral shoulder dislocation reduced and stabilized with glenohumeral K-wiring.

of the humerus head aiming toward the center of the humeral head and transfixing the shoulder joint in to the glenoid as shown in the upward direction and along the plane of scapula (directed 20 to 30 degrees posterior to coronal plane). The wire is also directed posteriorly considering the humerus retroversion and posterior placement of scapula.

Proximal Humerus Fractures

Proximal humeral fracture is one of the most frequent osteoporotic fractures in the elderly people, accounting for 6% of all fractures seen in accident and emergency departments.

Most proximal humeral fractures are undisplaced (85%) or minimally displaced and can be treated successfully nonoperatively. The remaining 15% displaced fracture may require surgery. The goal of fracture treatment is to get the fracture fragment to "move as a unit" at the earliest possible time to avoid stiffness. This can be achieved by percutaneous K-wire fixation or internal fixation with osseoaponeurotic stitches and PHILOS (Proximal Humerus Internal Locking System) plate osteosynthesis.

The number of fracture fragments, the displacement, and the dislocation indicate the severity and complexity of these fractures. Many times these fractures are amenable for closed reduction and K-wire fixation irrespective of the age. One must master the technique of closed reduction of two-part, three-part, and four-part fractures. The author strongly feels this comes with experience, understanding the biomechanics, the deforming forces, and how to neutralize and reduce the different parts like a jigsaw puzzle.

If one cannot anatomically reduce these fractures either by closed means or by limited open technique then we cannot proceed to threaded K-wire fixation.

The crux is the reduction and maintenance of the fracture fragments with K-wires or minimally invasive percutaneous plate osteosynthesis (MIPPO). One must master the technique of reduction and their concepts before fixation with K-wire. If one cannot reduce the fracture, then there is no hesitation to do open reduction and internal fixation with PHILOS plate, which in our center is less than 10%.

Percutaneous K-wire fixation is done by marking the site of deltoid insertion in the upper arm, and a skin incision is made 1 cm above the deltoid distal insertion. Starting from just above the site of deltoid insertion, threaded K-wires of 2.5 or 3 mm were inserted starting from the lateral cortex of upper shaft. The entry on the bone is usually double the distance of the height of the humeral head (**Fig. 7.11**). This is aimed toward the medial calcar in an oblique fashion at an angle of 60 to 70 degrees. The trick here is to start at 45-degree angle to make a mark on the bone and gently move the arm more parallel to the drill machine rather than moving the drilling machine more oblique to the shaft. This avoids frequent slippage on the humerus lateral cortex. Minimum two lateral to medial and one AP threaded K-wires were used to fix the fracture. One or two pins from greater tuberosity to medial shaft could also be done if necessary. One must avoid axillary nerve damage by following the surface marking for entry of K-wire from the shaft. Usually the nerve is at 5 cm below the acromion process. Too low entry can injure the radial nerve (**Fig. 7.12**). The biggest advantage of K-wire fixation is that it is a less invasive, less time consuming, least morbid procedure in fragile elderly patients and no second surgery like implant removal is necessary.

At the end of the procedure, the shoulder should be checked for full external and internal rotation in both AP and axillary view to evaluate the stability of the construct and to avoid protrusion of the pins into the joint.

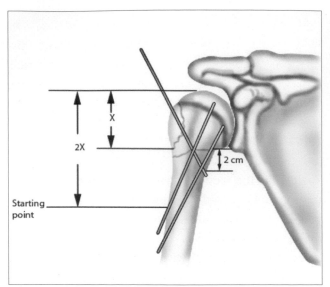

Fig. 7.11 Surface markings for K-wire entry.

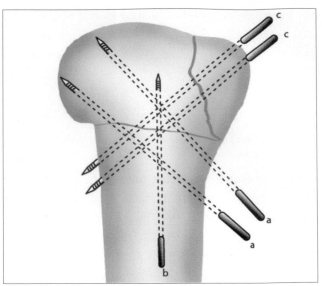

Fig. 7.12 Pictorial representation of the passage of K-wire in proximal humerus fracture.

Any catch on rotation or abduction indicates intra-articular penetration of K-wire. These K-wires are parked subchondrally on the head for better purchase. The best way to assess when the K-wire tip is closest to the articular margin in one particular position is by gently rotating 10 to 20 degrees on either side to look for joint penetration or the wire tip is moving away from the joint margin. The pins used to fix surgical neck fracture from the humeral shaft to head must be placed in the safe zone on the anterolateral cortex such that it avoids the radial and axillary nerves. The radial nerve is relatively protected if the pins are kept above the deltoid insertion. The axillary nerve is located an average of 5 cm distal to the acromion. Humeral retroversion is 25 to 30 degrees and the pin must be directed posteromedially to account for this angle.

Two-Part Surgical Neck of Humerus Fracture

This is reduced by gentle axial traction with forward flexion and abduction of 30 degrees, holding the elbow in 90-degree flexion with arm in 45-degree internal rotation. The distal fragment is pulled medially by the force of pectoralis major which can be neutralized by adducting the arm and by direct pressure over the distal fragment to correct the medial angulation. In obese patients, it will be easier to use a towel around the upper arm to pull the distal fragment laterally keeping the arm in adduction.

The first threaded K-wire is passed from the humerus shaft into the humerus head transfixing the fracture as discussed previously. While entering the shaft it may again re-displace medially because of the force used to enter with the wire. One should recheck the reduction before crossing the fracture site. Remanipulation may be necessary at this step. After positioning the first wire in good position along the medial calcar with anatomic reduction it is unlikely to get displaced while entering with the second wire. After positioning three-threaded K-wires subchondrally, a continuous fluoroscopy is done to check there is no puncturing of the articular surface in all directions.

In elderly patients with osteoporotic bone, these proximal humerus fractures are quite common. In closed manipulation by gentle forward flexion of 30 to 40 degrees, abduction of 30 to 40 degrees, and internal rotation of 45 degrees under C-arm control, one should check for acceptable reduction. Fine-tuning can be done at this stage to check for the desired position and try to achieve normal angle of neck shaft inclination (135 degrees). Percutaneous threaded K-wire should be used to prevent migration of K-wire into the chest wall. Two lateral K-wires are passed from the humeral shaft at the site of insertion of deltoid aiming toward the medial calcar of the head in an oblique fashion (60–70 degrees). This may be technically difficult to get in too oblique onto the shaft. One can start drilling at 45-degrees obliquity to make a mark in the bone and then slowly increase its obliquity by drilling almost parallel to the shaft, so that the distal part of the wire can enter the humeral head near the calcar.

Two anterolateral wires are passed in a similar fashion to enter the humeral head, which is normally retroverted at 30 degrees. The fixation in two planes with four wires can allow the whole of the proximal humerus to move as one unit for early range of motion and to prevent stiffness. Two- or three-threaded K-wires were passed from the humeral shaft to the humerus head and additional greater tuberosity K-wire from above to medial calcar shaft like a cross pin in special situations like gross osteoporosis and inadequate fixation.

In general, wire fixation from greater tuberosity is avoided as this jeopardizes early range of motion of shoulder because of deltoid tethering by the wire. We may use it rarely if additional fixation is necessary for stability. If K-wire from greater tuberosity is used, we tend to remove it early by 3 to 4 weeks to start passive range of motion to prevent stiffness.

Some of the threaded K-wires loosen by 3 to 4 weeks postoperatively, which warrants removal to prevent infection and pain. Patient should be warned about this possible problem. In general, the wire is removed at 4 to 5 weeks, and one may not wait for radiological evidence of healing in order to prevent stiffness.

Case Scenario 1

In a young man with good-quality bone with displaced neck of humerus fracture, closed manipulation, reduction, and percutaneous threaded K-wire fixation was done by maintaining the humerus valgus angle (**Fig. 7.13a, b**).

Case Scenario 2

Displaced neck of humerus fracture fixed with three threaded K-wires from shaft (**Fig. 7.14a–d**).

Case Scenario 3

Two-part surgical neck humerus (**Fig. 7.15a–o**). Here the distal fragment is adducted in AP view because of the pull of pectoralis major muscle, and in the axial view, the head is totally disconnected and retroverted with the shaft lying anteriorly. Closed manipulation was done with axial traction and arm in adduction; the distal fragment was pushed posteriorly and laterally so that the shaft displaces back, locks on to the head fragment, and swings the humerus head on its end to get normal alignment. Surface marking of the deltoid insertion was done. One centimeter above the deltoid insertion, the K-wires were inserted from the skin surface and on the shaft distally from double the distance of the humerus head aiming toward the inferior aspect of the head. Two lateral and one AP wires were passed to secure the humerus head.

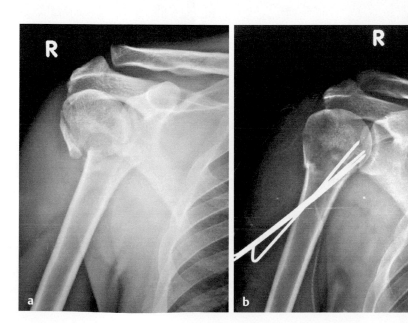

Fig. 7.13 (**a, b**) Anatomical reduction with maintenance of valgus angle that gives the best result with percuatneous k wire fixation.

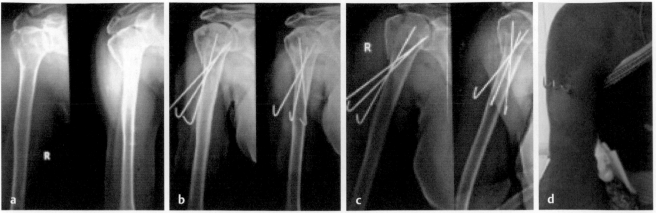

Fig. 7.14 **(a–d)** Two lateral and one anterolateral threaded K-wires were passed to fix the retroverted humeral head.

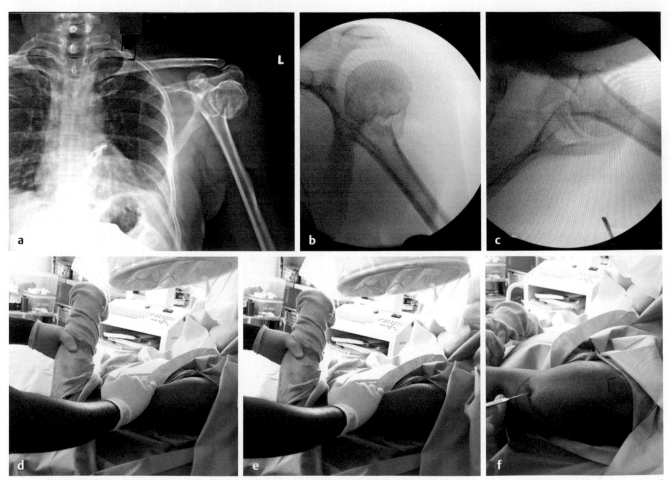

Fig. 7.15 **(a–f)** Methodology of closed reduction technique with percutaneous threaded K-wire fixation of two-part surgical neck humerus.

Case Scenario 4

Closed reduction and percutaneous K-wiring AP and axial views of two-part fracture (**Fig. 7.16a–c**).

Case Scenario 5

Totally displaced fracture neck of humerus with shaft displacing anteriorly and head lying posterior was

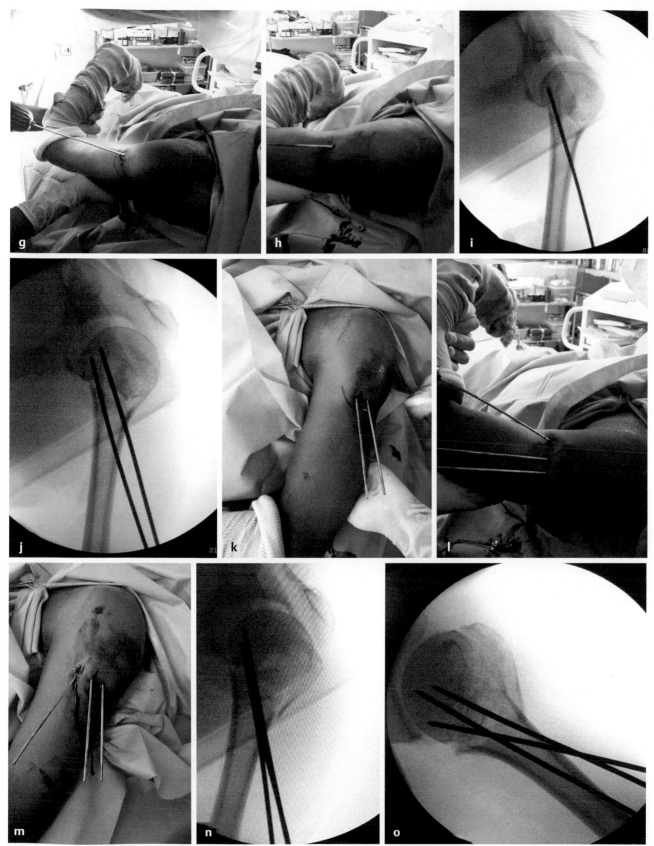

Fig. 7.15 *(Continued)* **(g–o)** Methodology of closed reduction technique with percutaneous threaded K-wire fixation of two-part surgical neck humerus.

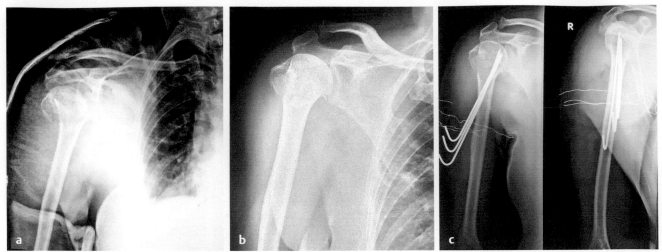

Fig. 7.16 **(a–c)** Figure demonstrating the closed reduction and percutaneous K-wiring anteroposterior (AP) and axial views.

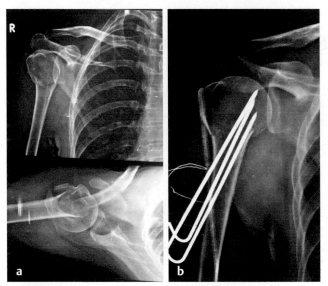

Fig. 7.17 **(a, b)** Fixation of the two-part fracture head of humerus.

reduced by manipulation and fixed with three percutaneous threaded K-wires (**Fig. 7.17a, b**).

Case Scenario 6

Here, the distal fragment was adducted because of the pull of pectoralis major. The shaft was displaced medially, anteriorly, and was rotated internally by the pull of pectoralis major. This force was minimized in closed manipulation by adducting the arm, flexing, and internally rotating to relax the pectoralis major muscle. With traction to the arm, lateral and downward forces were applied at the apex of the angulation for reduction and

the distal fragment was aligned to the humerus head. Once reduced, the humerus can be externally rotated gently to a neutral position such that the humeral shaft rotationally aligns with humeral head. The arm can be positioned at the side or in slight abduction, depending on the degree of varus of the humeral head. 2 lateral and 2 anterolateral wires were passed to fix the fracture. Good Functional outcome seen at the end of 4 months of follow up (**Fig. 7.18a–j**).

Case Scenario 7

Totally displaced fracture reduced and fixed with threaded K-wires from shaft and greater tuberosity because of osteoporosis (**Fig. 7.19a–f**).

Case Scenario 8

Two-part fracture surgical neck of humerus with anterior angulation (retroverted head) (**Fig. 7.20a–m**). In a low-velocity injury with fall on outstretched hand, a simple two-part fracture with minimal mediolateral displacement but with gross anterior angulation is not uncommon. A true axial view or a computed tomography (CT) scan will help us to identify this deformity. Here the distal fragment was moved anterior to the head of humerus resulting in anterior angulation and head more retroverted. This was manipulated by gentle axial traction by holding arm in 30-degree forward flexion, 30-degree abduction, and 45-degree internal rotation with elbow flexed to 90 degree to distract the

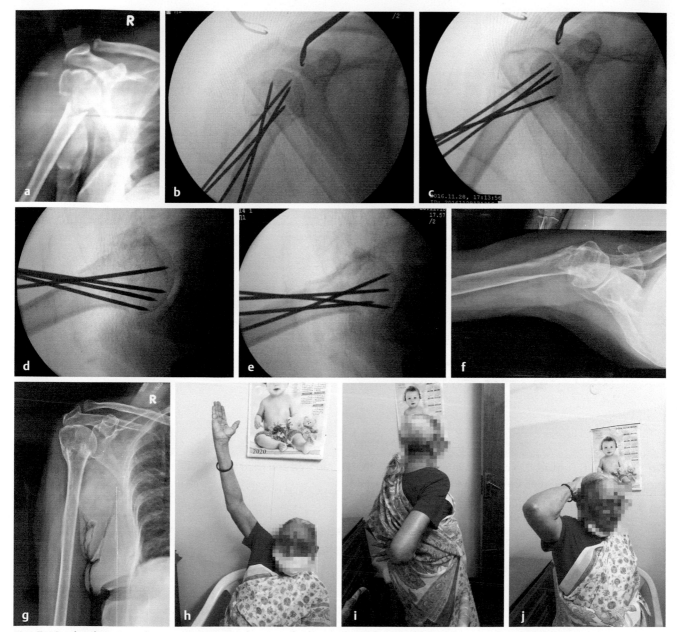

Fig. 7.18 **(a–j)** Patient demonstrating good range of movements following healed fracture fixation.

fracture. A direct anterior pressure over the distal shaft fragment at the site of angulation reduced the fracture and the head swung anteriorly correcting the excessive retroversion. Once the head was on the humerus shaft, the axial force was reduced to lock in that position and then the head and shaft fragment would move as one unit. In the conventional manner three percutaneous threaded guidewires were passed in good position parking subchondrally.

Case Scenario 9

Reverse oblique neck of humerus fracture (**Fig. 7.21a–g**). A threaded K-wire was introduced into the head to maintain the normal head shaft angle and to control rotation like a joystick. Subsequently, the convention K-wires were passed in the routine manner aiming at the thick medial calcar area in the inferior aspect of the humerus head. Once three K-wires secured the fracture in anatomical position, the joystick head wire was removed.

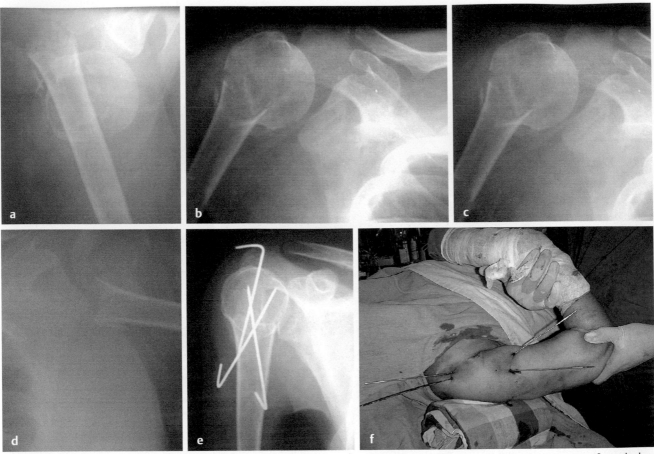

Fig. 7.19 (a–f) Displaced two-part fracture with osteoporosis, reduced and fixed with threaded K-wires, starting from below through the shaft and then from the greater tuberosity.

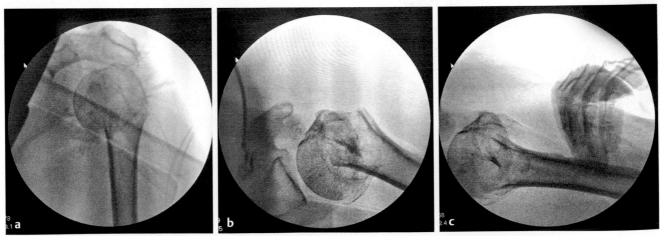

Fig. 7.20 (a–c) Closed reduction and sequential K-wire placement of surgical neck of humerus fracture.

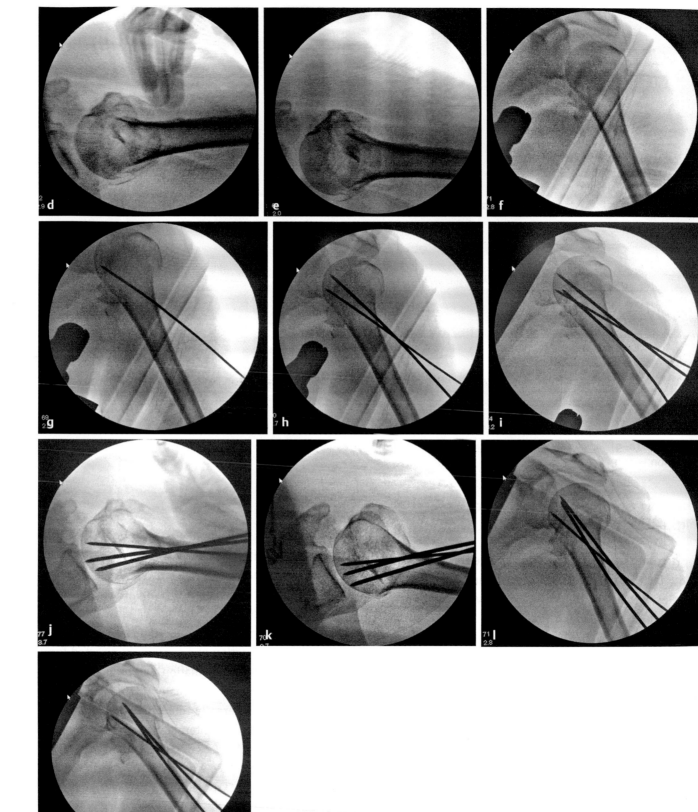

antegra[...]
ture gre[...]
fragmen[...]
Only su[...]
complet[...]

Case S[...]

This wa[...]
tion in 3[...]
forearm[...]
humeral[...]
threaded[...]

Fig. 7.20 *(Continued)* **(d–m)** Closed reduction and sequential K-wire placement of surgical neck of humerus fracture.

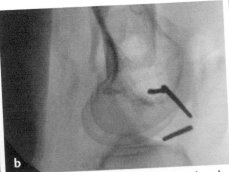
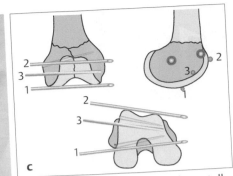

Fig. 10.2 **(a–c)** Placement of two K-wires, one at the joint level by free-hand and another at trochlear level under the patella. The third K-wire was introduced intraosseously parallel to the above wires 2 cm above the joint level and at the junction of anterior one-third and posterior two-thirds of the femoral condyle.

Positioning of Locking Plate

Locking plates, commonly used, have a hole on either ends for K-wire insertion for perfect positioning in vivo. For example, when a femoral buttress locking plate is used by minimally invasive plate osteosynthesis technique, the proximal placement is secured close to the bone by a K-wire, and distal placement on the shaft is centralized by another K-wire at the distal end. Subsequently, the osteosynthesis with screws is completed.

The K-wire is used in a similar fashion in less-invasive stabilization system (LISS) for the distal femur LISS locking plate, proximal humerus internal locking system (PHILOS), and all types of locking plates (**Fig. 10.3**).

Pediatric Open Fracture Femur

A child with grade 3 open fracture over the medial aspect of the distal thigh with severe comminution was treated by multiple cross K-wires passed from the metaphyseal area (without entering the physis) into the diaphysis of femur. This was protected by above-knee cast with a window for regular wound inspection and dressing. Slight bent in the K-wire was seen in 3 weeks' follow-up because of loose above-knee plaster of Paris (POP) cast. The final X-ray after 2 months showed adequate callus and healing in good alignment (**Fig. 10.4a–g**).

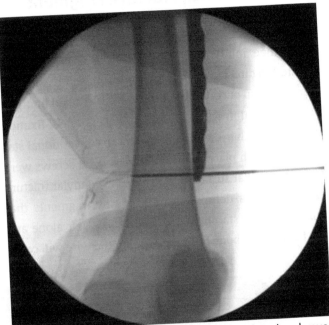

Fig. 10.3 Proximal femur locking plate placed submuscularly was secured to the shaft in the center of anteroposterior plane by a K-wire through the hole in the plate.

Supracondylar Fracture Distal Femur in a Child

The posteriorly displaced supracondylar fracture femur in a 9-year-old child with varus deformity was corrected by closed manipulation and reduction under anesthesia by traction and valgus with extension force on the distal

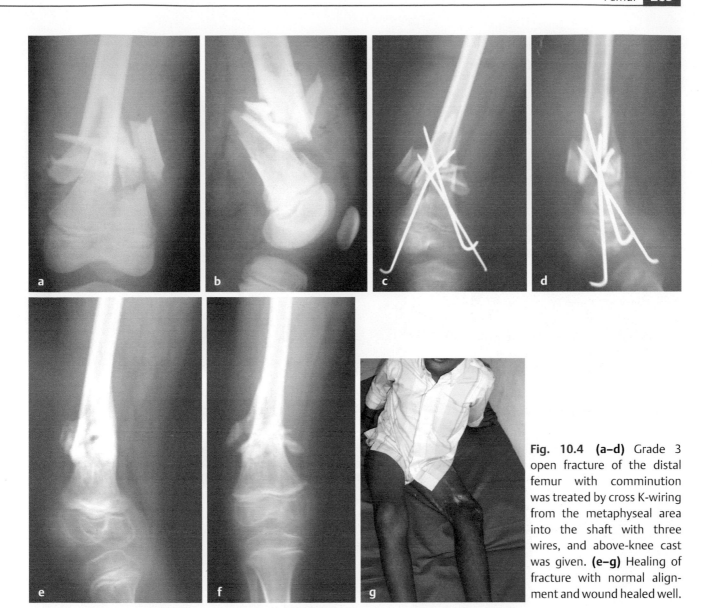

Fig. 10.4 (a–d) Grade 3 open fracture of the distal femur with comminution was treated by cross K-wiring from the metaphyseal area into the shaft with three wires, and above-knee cast was given. **(e–g)** Healing of fracture with normal alignment and wound healed well.

fragment (**Fig. 10.5a–j**). The reduction was maintained and fixed with two cross K-wires of 2.5 mm from medial and lateral condyle of femur starting at the metaphysis just above the physis level. An above-knee POP cast was applied. The K-wire and POP cast was removed at the end of 5 weeks. Graded mobilization and weight-bearing activities were started.

Periprosthetic Fracture Shaft of Femur

Patient with cemented bipolar hemiarthroplasty had periprosthetic fracture involving the shaft of femur

(**Fig. 10.6a–g**). Long spiral comminution fracture with no loosening of prosthesis was treated by anatomical reduction by securing and matching the spiral segments and was stabilized with temporary K-wires perpendicular to the plane, giving room for the placement of proximal femur locking plate. The locking plate was positioned correctly and secured with K-wire at the lower end of the plate. Stainless steel cerclage wire was used to stabilize the spiral fracture, and locking screws were used to secure the plate missing the femoral prosthesis in the proximal part. When stable fixation was obtained, K-wires were removed.

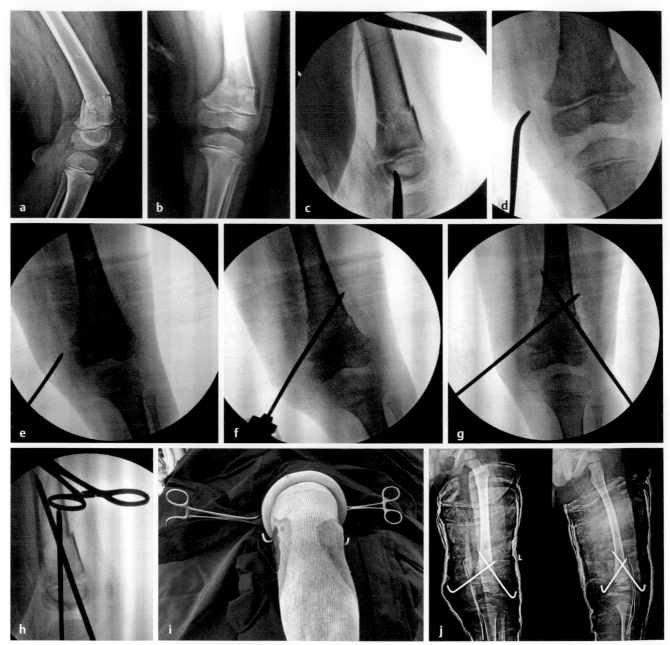

Fig. 10.5 **(a–j)** Supracondylar femur fracture reduced and fixed with two cross K-wires.

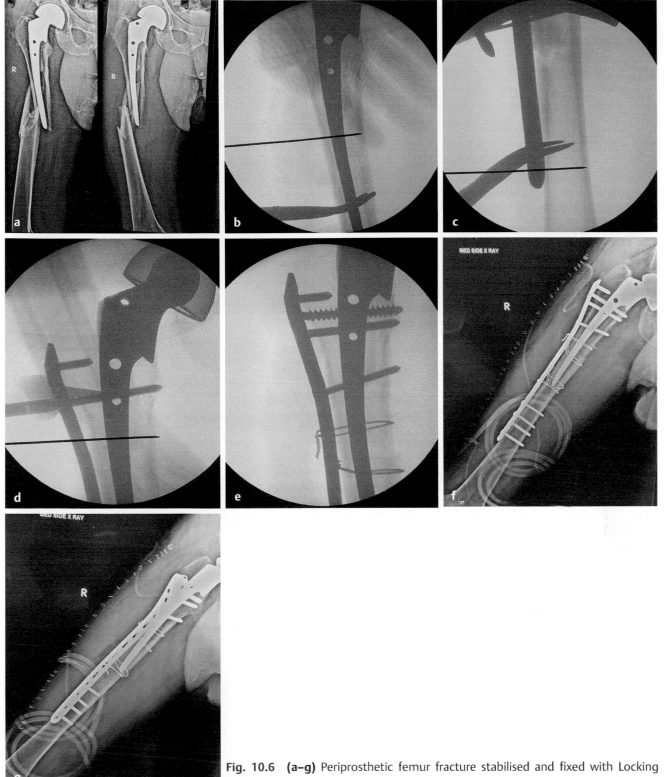

Fig. 10.6 (a–g) Periprosthetic femur fracture stabilised and fixed with Locking plate.

K-Wires in Pathological Fracture of Femur (Osteopetrosis)

Osteopetrosis is also known as the marble bone disease. It is rightly called so because the bone is rock solid with no medullary canal in the long bone in this condition. In an osteopetrosis patient as the bone is tough, drilling becomes a surgical challenge. Tough bone easily breaks the drill bits during the procedure. This patient had pathological subtrochanteric femur fracture with no medullary canal. A 4.5-mm drill bit was used to enter the piriformis fossa. With lot of difficulty, the medullary canal was opened. Once centered in anteroposterior and lateral image intensifier pictures, a thick 4-mm K-wire was used to create a tract in the so-called medullary canal area slowly. This was preferred, as the K-wire is flexible and does not break like the drill bit. Again, after entering every centimeter it was rinsed with saline to dissipate the heat. K-wire could hardly be crossed beyond the fracture for 4 cm and it was left alone. This procedure simply worked like a transfixation thick K-wire across the fracture so that it may not displace further. Because this fixation was flimsy, patient was kept in bed with skin traction for 6 weeks and non–weight bearing for 3 months. Eventually fracture healed well and patient came with similar pathological fracture in the opposite femur undisplaced and again the same method was used successfully to heal the other fracture (**Fig. 10.7a, b**).

Chronic Lower Femoral Epiphyseal Separation

Chronic lower femoral epiphyseal separation is a rare occurrence in a 9-year-old girl who had a trivial trauma 2 months back that was treated initially like a sprain using local native method. She presented late to us with difficulty in weight bearing and walking. She was having a condition called "congenital insensitivity to pain." The X-ray showed widening of physis with varus shift and new bone formation along the metaphyseal area indicating the chronic nature. Because of insensitivity to pain, the physeal injury behaved like a neuropathic fracture with inability to heal. On examination under anesthesia, the lower femoral epiphysis was moving separately with varus and valgus stress. This was stabilized with cross K-wires from medial and lateral condyles after obtaining maximum correction of alignment by closed manipulation as shown in **Fig. 10.8a–d**. An additional above-knee POP cast was given.

"T"-Type Physeal Fracture Distal End Femur

This is a rare type of physeal fracture with anterior displacement of distal femoral physis (**Fig. 10.9a–o**). The CT scan depicts the physeal fracture line as "T" shaped with complete physeal line fracture with displacement, and the intercondylar split which was undisplaced. Closed

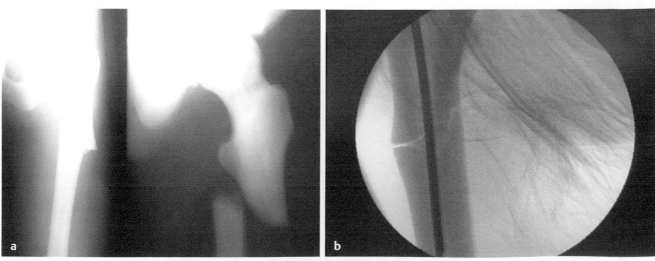

Fig. 10.7 **(a, b)** Osteopetrosis treated with 4-mm-thick intramedullary K-wire negotiated with difficulty.

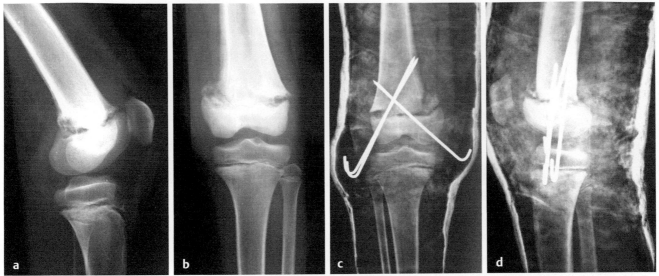

Fig. 10.8 (a–d) Lower femoral epiphyseal separation with instability was treated with closed manipulation and pinning with minimum three K-wires from epiphysis to metaphyseal cortex.

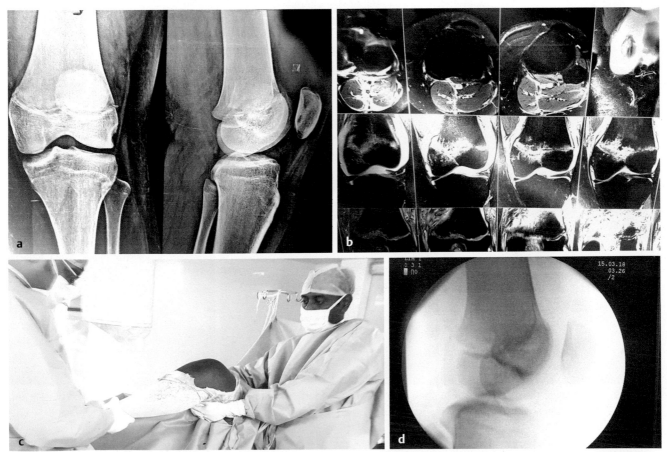

Fig. 10.9 (a–d) T-type physeal fracture distal end of femur reduced and fixed with transphyseal cross K-wire and epiphyseal cannulated screw fixation. *(Continued)*

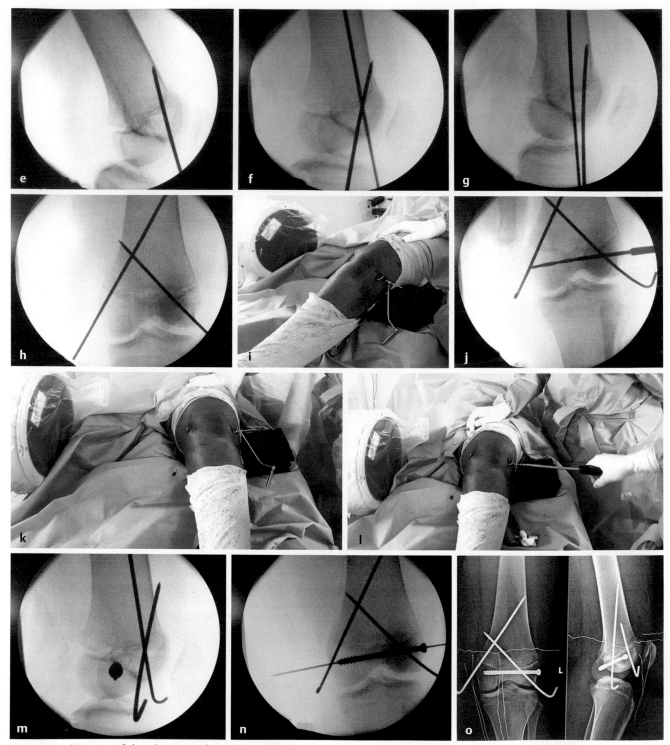

Fig. 10.9 (*Continued*) **(e–o)** T-type physeal fracture distal end of femur reduced and fixed with transphyseal cross K-wire and epiphyseal cannulated screw fixation.

reduction with traction in flexion of the knee and counterpressure at thigh to stabilize femur was able to reduce the fracture which was hyperextended. Two cross thick K-wires were passed from medial and lateral condyles across the physeal line into the opposite far cortex of distal femoral shaft as shown in **Fig. 10.9h**. A guidewire was passed from lateral to medial direction just below and parallel to the physeal line fixing the intercondylar epiphysis fracture in good position. A cannulated 7 mm partially threaded cancellous screw was used to fix the fracture with anatomical reduction. An above-knee cast was given in the postoperative period of 4 weeks and subsequently the K-wires were removed.

Segmental Bone Loss—Structural Graft Fillers

Huge segmental bone loss due to trauma or infection resulting in excision of bone, or tumor resection, needs filling up of the void with segmental intercalary structural bone graft. Usually bone defects within 7 cm can be bridged with autologous iliac crest graft or fibula strut graft or allografts. Bone defects more than 7 cm may require bone transport procedure. These grafts can be fixed to the host bone by transosseous K-wires or screw fixation depending on the size and strength. The X-ray shows defect in the lower third femur with plate in situ. The tricortical iliac crest graft is fixed proximally with two transfixation K-wires in different planes after jamming the graft into the host bone, and distally the graft is secured in place to the host bone with a cancellous screw (**Fig. 10.10a–e**).

Infected Open Fracture Distal Femur with Gap Defect

A case of Gustilo type 3b open fracture was treated initially with distal femur locking plate that got infected.

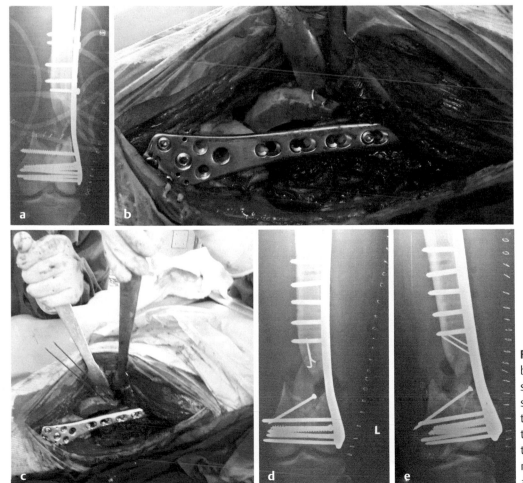

Fig. 10.10 (a–e) Segmental bone defect filled with structural iliac crest graft secured proximally within the bone trough with two transfixation K-wires. Distally the graft is impacted into the metaphysis and secured with a cancellous screw.

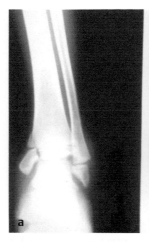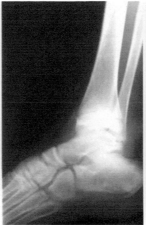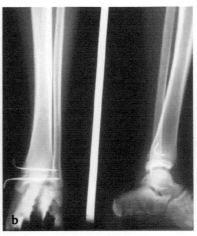

Fig. 13.12 (a, b) Salter-Harris type 4 fracture anatomically reduced and fixed with transverse K-wires through the metaphysis and epiphysis without crossing the physis.

Pilon Fracture

The first step in treating the pilon fracture was to restore the length of the fibula that can be easily obtained in a swollen leg with intramedullary K-wire fixation as shown in **Fig. 13.13a, b**. The fragmented metaphyseal area was anatomically restored for articular surface congruity. This was maintained by subchondral K-wire fixation. Additional lag screws can be added if fragments are large. In **Fig. 13.13** one AP K-wire and another K-wire from medial malleolus to metaphyseal site were driven to maintain the reduction. The metaphyseodiaphyseal stabilization was done with joint spanning external fixator with good alignment of the leg using the principle of ligamentotaxis. These percutaneous K-wires were kept for 6 weeks until fracture consolidates, but the fixator was maintained for 3 months.

Transcalcaneal Tibiotalar K-Wiring

Transcalcaneal tibiotalar K-wiring is indicated in conditions such as high-grade ankle fractures with unstable fracture—dislocations of ankle, global instability of ankle in high-velocity injuries, open fracture dislocations of the ankle with severe soft tissue damage, or contaminants and mild talar tilt or shift even after conventional plate and screw fixation as an additional rescue procedure to give congruent ankle joint. This procedure can be added even after fixing a bimalleolar fracture if the surgeon is not happy about congruous reduction in both AP and lateral view pictures, especially in lateral view if one can demonstrate posterior subluxation in plantarflexion and dorsiflexion of the ankle causing congruous reduction. This is a foolproof technique used to maintain the congruity of the joint for 6 weeks. This procedure can be considered as a salvage procedure in very unstable ankle fractures in patients with uncontrolled diabetes; poor skin conditions due to blisters; pedal edema; and precarious circulation to the limb, postphlebitic limb, neuropathic foot and ankle. A 4-mm thick K-wire or a 5mm Steinmann pin was used for this procedure. Author prefers K-wire because it causes less damage to the chondral surface. An additional below-knee supportive splint or plaster of Paris (POP) slab is necessary.

The ankle joint is reduced and checked using image intensifier. Skin markings are made by drawing a line centering the ankle joint in AP and lateral views. The line bisecting on the plantar aspect of the heel is the site of insertion of K-wire. A skin incision was made and artery forceps was used to dissect bluntly and free tissues up to plantar aspect of the calcaneum. K-wire was drilled with a power driver checking in AP and lateral views of C-arm scan while crossing the subtalar joint and talotibial joint keeping the foot in neutral plantigrade position. It is important to cross the articular surfaces in a single attempt in order to avoid unnecessary chondral injury. Once crossed, the pin can be advanced up to 4 to 5 cm and the wire is left outside for easy removal later. The pin wound is irrigated with normal saline and a Jelonet dressing is given.

The advantages include minimal invasiveness, least soft tissue damage, technical easiness, minimal chance

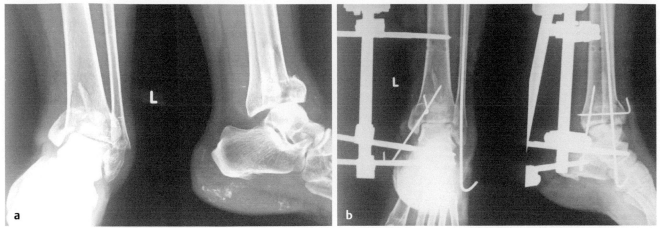

Fig. 13.13 (a, b) Pilon fracture reduced and fixed with lateral malleolus intramedullary K-wire, fragment specific joint reduction K-wire and sparing external fixator.

of infection, and no serious surgical wound site complications unlike in plate fixation such as skin breakdown, infection, or exposed implant, etc., easy for plastic surgical procedure in reconstructive surgery (unlike external fixation) and implant exit after fracture healing in 8 to 12 weeks' time. This procedure is ideal in these selective unstable ankle fractures, which is patient and surgeon-friendly considering the high-grade injury to the soft tissues and bone.

There is only theoretical risk of articular cartilage damage due to this pin fixation as this causes less than 5% of chondral surface injury. The risk of ankle stiffness due to temporary pin fixation is negligible and more dictated by associated soft tissue scarring or chondral damage in open injuries.

Case Scenarios

Case Scenario 1: Comminuted Pilon Fracture

A 44-year-old man sustained injury to his right ankle and X-ray showed severely unstable comminuted pilon fracture. First, the lateral malleolus was fixed to get the ankle out of length and alignment, and by a K-wire the medial malleolus was aligned temporarily for articular congruity, and subsequently fixed with the malleolar screw. After fixation the ankle joint was still unstable because of global capsular disruption. Hence, fixation by percutaneous transcalcaneal 5-mm and 4-mm-thick two

K-wires were done (**Fig. 13.14a–g**). The ankle joint was found stable and congruity was maintained.

Case Scenario 2: Open Fracture Dislocation Ankle

A 55-year-old man had severe open ankle fracture dislocation with stripping of the soft tissues from lower third of the tibia. After thorough wound debridement, the ankle joint was relocated and **Fig. 13.15a–i** shows comminuted medial malleolus fracture. This was fixed with cancellous screw with washer and additional K-wire for stability. Even after this fixation, the joint was subluxing because of the global instability from capsular tear. A transcalcaneal thick K-wire was used to correct this instability. A 6-month postsurgery clinical picture showed good end result.

Case Scenario 3: Crush Injury Foot and Open Ankle Fracture Dislocation

A 52-year-old man had road traffic accident with severe crush injury to the right foot. X-ray of the right ankle with foot showed ankle fracture dislocation with multiple metatarsal fractures with autoamputated great toe at metatarsal level (**Fig. 13.16a–e**). Thorough wash and wound debridement was done with first metatarsal terminalization. The dislocated joint was relocated and a percutaneous transcalcaneal 4-mm-thick K-wire joint transfixation was done. There was a loss of bone

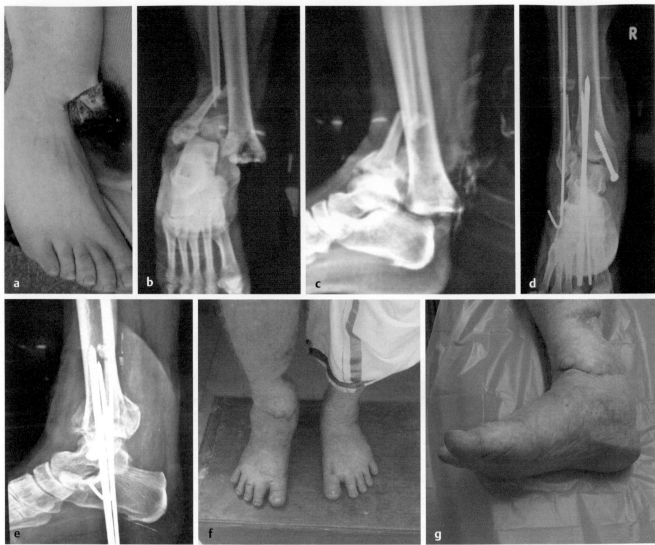

Fig. 13.14 (a–g) Open pilon fracture dislocation after debridement was reduced and fixed with intramedullary K-wire for fibula fracture and transarticular transcalcaneal thick K-wire fixation for ankle mortise. Good end result.

from medial malleolus and the remaining fragment of medial malleolus was fixed with a transverse screw. Transcalcaneal ankle pinning is a much easier option of stabilization than external fixator which is rather cumbersome for the plastic surgeons to work and is not patient friendly. Ankle joint stability was obtained with single transcalcaneal thick K-wire and external below-knee synthetic splint. If the pin stabilization is inadequate, one more transcalcaneal thick K-wire can be added for more rotational stability. A 6-weeks postsurgery shows a plantigrade foot with healed split skin graft.

Case Scenario 4: Malunited Fracture Dislocation Ankle (Fig. 13.17a–d)

A 9-month-old malunited fracture dislocation of ankle with posterolateral displacement was noted. Open reduction with osteotomy of posterolateral malunited fragment of tibia and malunited fibula was done. By medial approach, the soft tissues in the medial gutter were cleared. The fibula length was regained, reduced, and fixed with intramedullary rush nail with bone grafting. The plate osteosynthesis of posterior fragment was

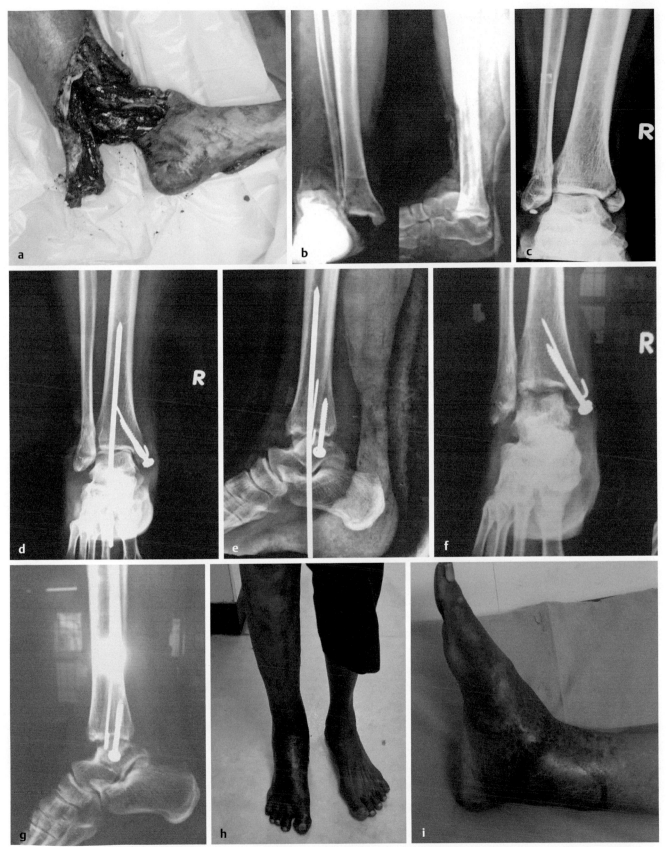

Fig. 13.15 **(a–i)** Open fracture dislocation ankle was stabilized by transcalcaneal thick K-wire and screw fixation. We prefer 3- or 4-mm-thick K-wire than Steinmann pin as it is less damaging to articular surface and the final clinical picture as shown.

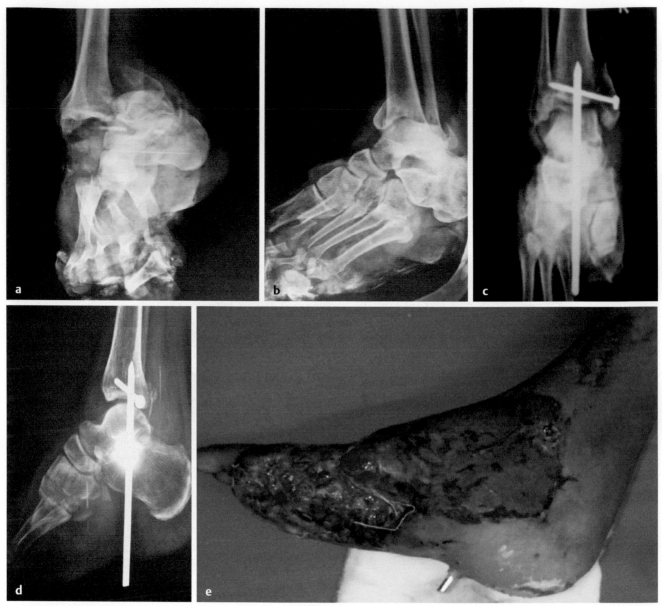

Fig. 13.16 (a–e) Crush injury to foot and ankle with dislocation and loss of bones treated by transarticular transcalcaneal K-wire and screw fixation as shown with the final picture after plastic surgery.

done with bone grafting. An additional transcalcaneal 4-mm-thick K-wire was passed across the ankle joint to maintain the reduction, to neutralize the deforming force, and to keep the joint congruency. Below-knee cast was given for a period of 6 weeks and subsequently K-wire was removed. Fracture healed completely and the patient was fully mobile independently at the end of 3 months.

Tibiocalcaneal Stabilization

Open fracture dislocation of the talus with loss of bone from the body of talus required temporary stabilization of tibiocalcaneal joint with a transfixation thick K-wire after debridement and excision of dead, loose fragments of the remaining talus. A 4-mm-thick K-wire was passed through plantar aspect of the midcalcaneum, a point in

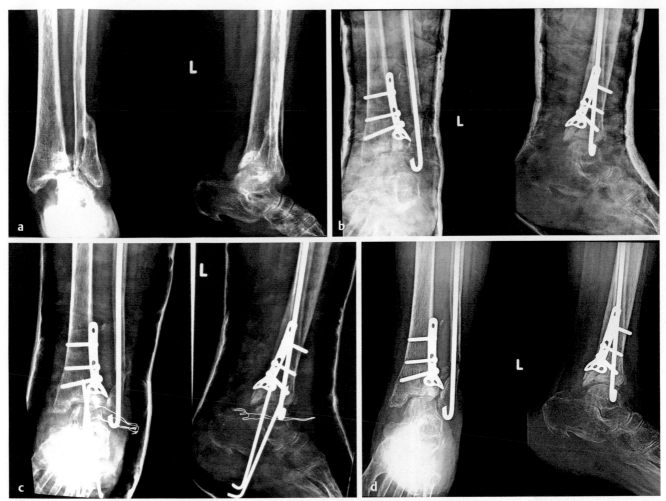

Fig. 13.17 **(a–d)** Malunited fracture dislocation of ankle with posterolateral displacement.

the anterior aspect of ball of the heel centering in lateral view toward the center of the ankle joint. A plantar skin incision was made, and artery forceps were used to spread the tissues and feel the plantar aspect of the calcaneum. K-wire was introduced into the calcaneum and tibia as shown in **Fig. 13.18a–d**. This was a temporary solution until the wound was managed and later on went in for tibiocalcaneal fusion. This procedure is less time consuming, less expensive, easy to perform plastic surgery, and patient friendly. Sometimes two thick wires were used to give rotational stability. A similar case scenario is shown in **Fig. 13.19a–d**.

Similar procedure was done for correction of severe talipes equinovarus deformity when talectomy was done in a child, as in cerebral palsy patient and neglected clubfoot patient.

Supramalleolar Osteotomy for Deformity Correction

A 14-year-old child had progressive valgus deformity following foot and ankle injury with soft tissue loss on the medial aspect. This led to growth disturbance of the distal tibial physis because of imbalance in the foot muscles and the nature of trauma. The child had fibula osteotomy, dome osteotomy of the distal tibia, and the ankle joint was made parallel to the floor. The corrected position was fixed with two parallel K-wires from medial malleolus as shown in **Fig. 13.20a–j**. Tendon balancing procedure was done and below-knee cast was given for 6 weeks. Then the K-wires were removed at 6 weeks and additional POP cast was given for 3 weeks period.

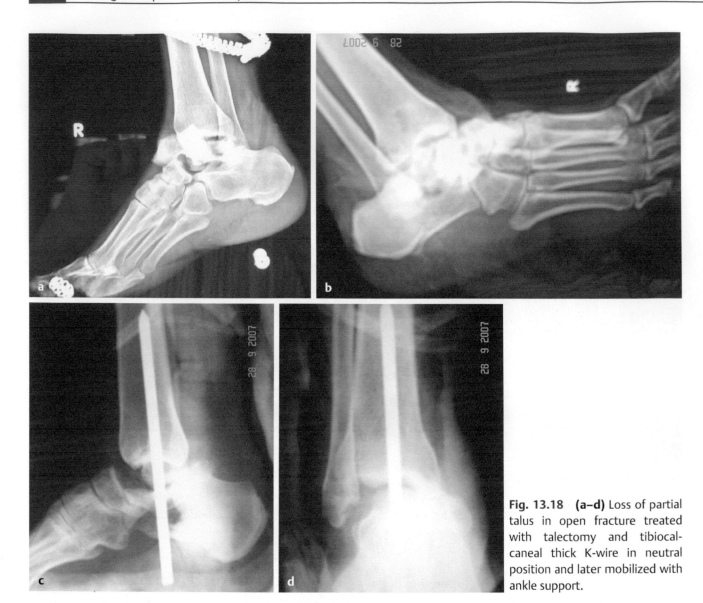

Fig. 13.18 (a–d) Loss of partial talus in open fracture treated with talectomy and tibiocalcaneal thick K-wire in neutral position and later mobilized with ankle support.

Fig. 13.19 (a–d) Open unstable ankle subluxation because of extensive soft tissue damage required some stability at ankle until the plastic surgical procedures are done. Here transcalcaneal 4-mm-thick K-wire was used to prevent subluxation of ankle instead of an external fixator.

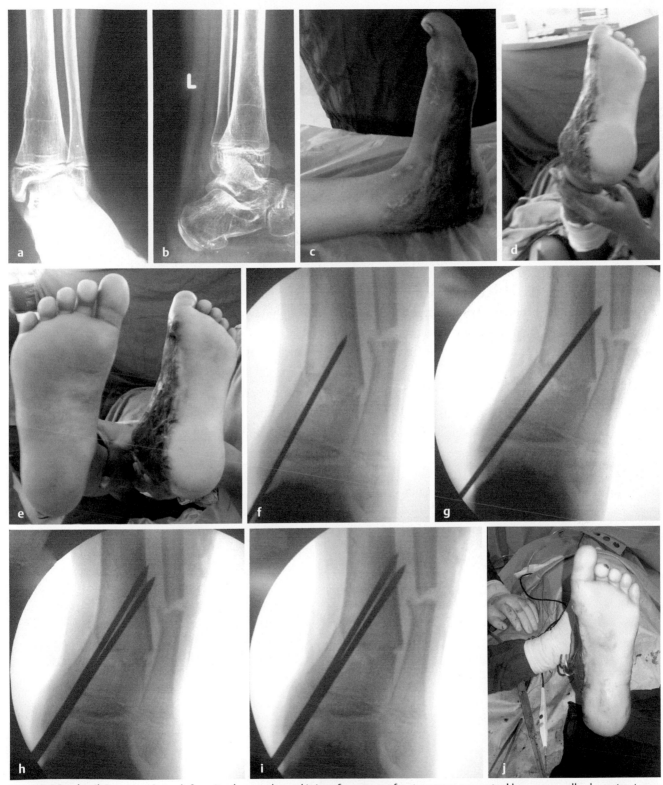

Fig. 13.20 (a–j) Severe valgus deformity due to physeal injury from open fracture was corrected by supramalleolar osteotomy of tibia and fibula. Percutaneous two parallel K-wires through medial malleolus holding the osteotomy was done to stabilize with accurate correction and the clinical picture shows the deformity well corrected.

14 Foot

Hindfoot

Subtalar Joint Depression-Type Fracture

Primary joint depression-type fracture without gross displacement of the major fragments is amenable for treatment with closed percutaneous reduction techniques. The maintenance of the reduced fragments is possible with percutaneous subchondral horizontal K-wires along the posterior subtalar joint. If major displacements are present, supplementary plate fixation may be necessary.

Case Scenario 1

Subtalar Joint depression type fracture due to fall from height.

Fig. 14.1a–c depicts the subtalar joint depression with a step that is elevated and maintained by a lateromedial K-wire insertion with image intensifier control.

Case Scenario 2

X-ray and computed tomography (CT) scan picture of calcaneum with splay out of the subtalar joint and depression.

Fig. 14.2a–d shows the X-ray and CT scan picture of calcaneum with splay out of the subtalar joint and depression. This is elevated and reduced with a thick K-wire passed under image intensifier control, using it as a joystick. A pointed reduction clamp around the calcaneum is applied with a longitudinal traction. The final

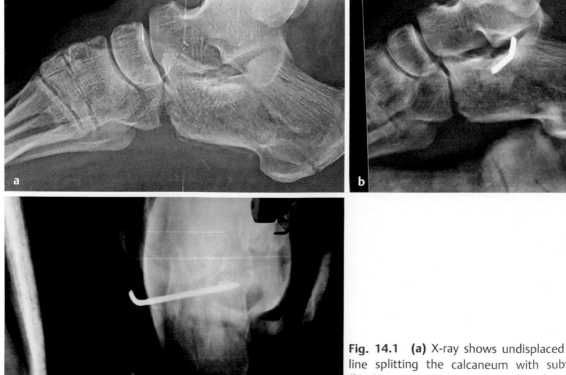

Fig. 14.1 (a) X-ray shows undisplaced primary fracture line splitting the calcaneum with subtalar depression. (b, c) Using K-wire as a joystick the depression is elevated and subchondral transverse K-wire fixation is done.

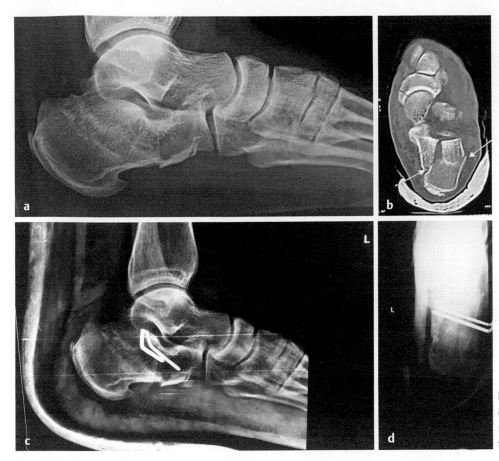

Fig. 14.2 (a–d) Split with depression of subtalar joint is reduced and maintained with two percutaneous K-wires.

reduced position is maintained with two percutaneous K-wires passed subchondrally from lateral aspect to medial cortex of calcaneum.

Case Scenario 3

Osteoporotic joint depression-type calcaneal fracture. An 80-year-old severely osteoporotic woman presents with joint depression fracture that is reduced by closed manipulation and reduction by thick K-wire used as a joystick to lift the subtalar depressed fragment to the maximum. This is maintained by percutaneous K-wires, as shown in **Fig. 14.3a–d** by passing subchondrally near the subtalar joint from posterolateral to anteromedial calcaneum transfixing the major fracture. Because it is osteoporotic compression fracture, the elevation may not be achieved to a great extent, but advantage of this simple fixation is to mobilize the subtalar and ankle joints from day 1 without much pain (as whole calcaneum moves as one unit) so as to mold the joint for congruency and movement.

Case Scenario 4

Comminuted calcaneal fracture. Severely comminuted fracture involving subtalar joint is treated by open reduction and internal fixation with K-wires and calcaneum plate. The subtalar joint is elevated, and lateral wall is closed to maintain the height and fixed with multiple K-wires, cut closed to the bone and buried to keep it in position. The major fragments are stabilized with calcaneal plate and screw in the conventional manner (**Fig. 14.4a, b**).

Calcaneum Tongue-Type Fracture

Case Scenario 1

According to Essex Lopresti classification, this tongue type of fracture is reduced by using a thick K-wire passed from the posterior calcaneal tuberosity in an oblique fashion and the upper fragment is levered down to reduce at the subtalar joint level and at the same time

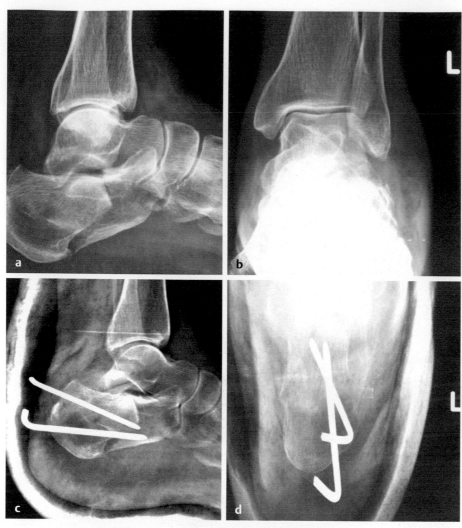

Fig. 14.3 (a–d) Percutaneous K-wire is passed from postero-lateral calcaneum to lift the subtalar fragment as much as possible, but because of severe osteoporosis, this is only partially achieved and accepted. The fragments are further stabilized with transfixation K-wire for early mobilization of subtalar joint without much pain and for proper molding.

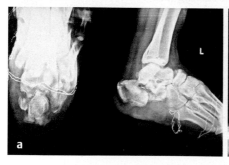

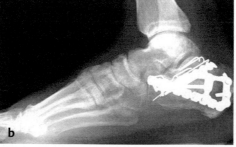

Fig. 14.4 (a, b) Young man with subtalar joint depression fracture that is elevated and fixed with multiple K-wires and plate-screw fixation.

pointed reduction clamp is used to correct the splay out and to keep in neutral alignment of hindfoot. Once subtalar congruent reduction is obtained, a percutaneous cannulated cancellous screw is inserted from postero-lateral calcaneal tuberosity to anteromedial sustentaculum tali fragment through the positioning of K-wire (**Fig. 14.5a–o**).

Case Scenario 2

Displaced tongue-type fracture can be reduced anatomically by plantar flexing in order to reduce the pull of tendoachilles and by applying a pointed reduction clamp. A K-wire is passed from the posterior tuberosity into the plantar fragment in desired position, perpendicular to the fracture pattern. The advantage of

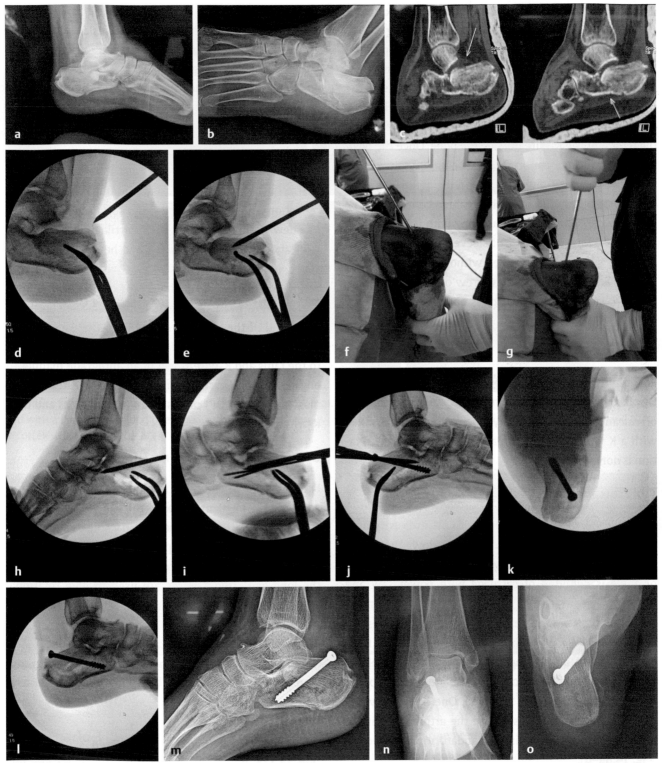

Fig. 14.5 **(a–o)** According to Essex Lopresti classification, this tongue type of fracture is reduced by using a thick K-wire that is passed from the posterior calcaneal tuberosity in an oblique fashion and the upper fragment is levered down to reduce at the subtalar joint level and at the same time pointed reduction clamp is used to correct the splay out and to keep in neutral alignment of hindfoot. Once subtalar congruent reduction is obtained a percutaneous cannulated cancellous screw is inserted from posterolateral calcaneal tuberosity to anteromedial sustentaculum tali fragment through the positioning K-wire.

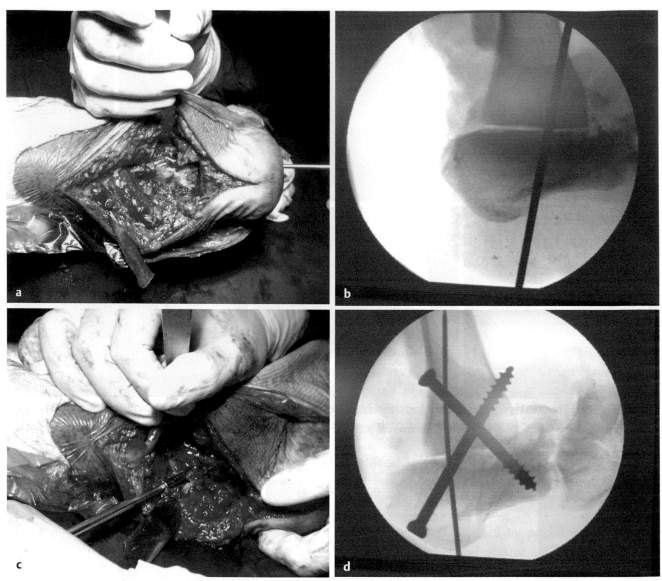

Fig. 14.8 (a–d) Posterior approach to the tibiocalcaneal fusion is done after matching the denuded surface on tibia and calcaneum transfixing in good position using a K-wire. Cross lag screws were applied to make it stable. Final tightening for lag effect at arthrodesis site was done after removing the K-wire.

The open wound is debrided, and the talonavicular joint is reduced anatomically and stabilized with two percutaneous K-wires passing from anteromedial aspect through the navicular bone into the talus. Stable reduction is achieved and the wound is primarily closed. An below-knee slab is given for 6 weeks.

Subtalar Dislocation (Fig. 14.16a–d)

Twisting injury to the foot resulting in isolated subtalar dislocation with whole foot supinated and adducted.

This is reduced by closed manipulation under anesthesia and stabilized with 3-mm transcalcaneal K-wire from the plantar aspect of sole, transfixing the talocalcaneal joint in congruent reduction.

Subtalar and Talonavicular Dislocation (Fig. 14.17a–h)

This combination is uncommon and happened due to forceful twisting of the ankle. Here with traction and direct pull-push technique the dislocation is reduced.

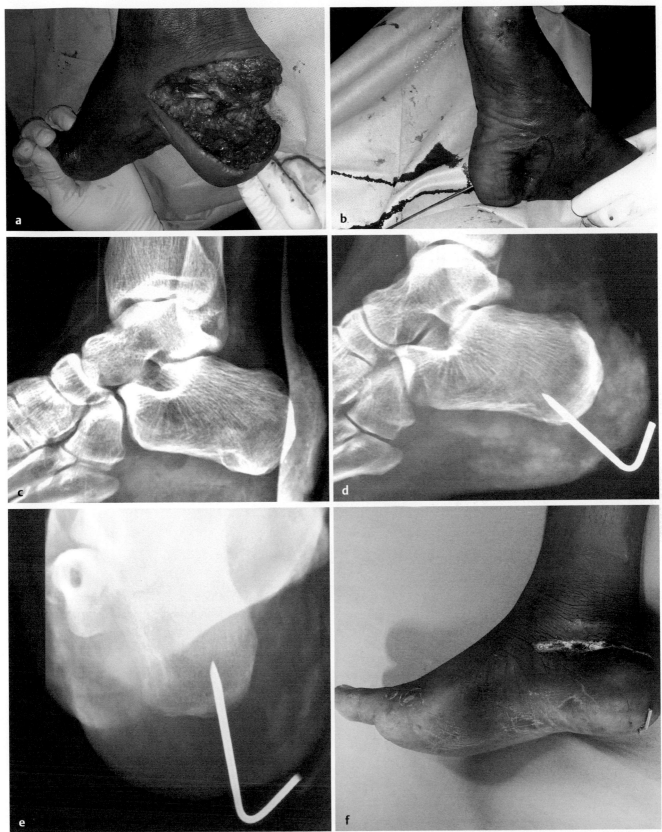

Fig. 14.9 (a–f) Heel flap avulsion is stabilized with a calcaneal K-wire to maintain the position and loose sutures applied for atraumatic surgery.

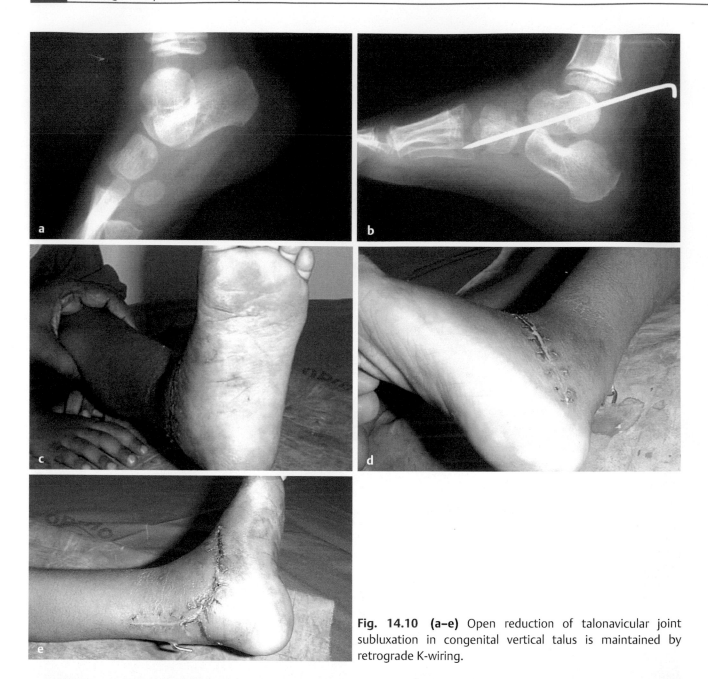

Fig. 14.10 (a–e) Open reduction of talonavicular joint subluxation in congenital vertical talus is maintained by retrograde K-wiring.

Fig. 14.11   (a–d) Two K-wires are used to transfix the fracture and to give rotational stability.

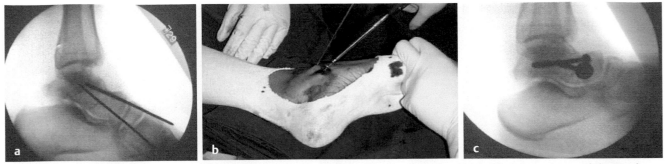

Fig. 14.12   **(a–c)** Cannulated cancellous screws are used to fix the fracture by using K-wire for temporary stability and as a guide.

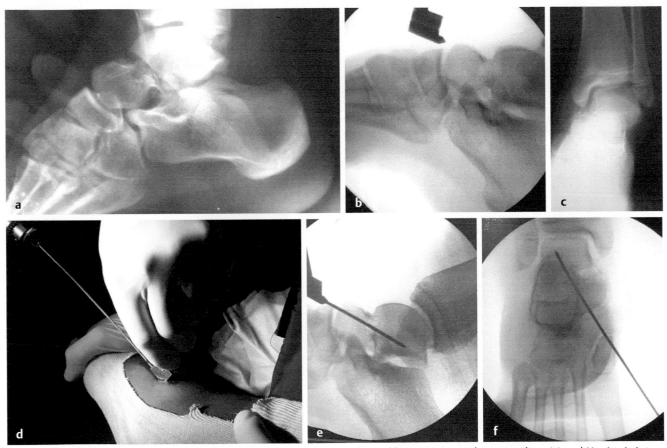

Fig. 14.13   **(a–c)** After closed reduction, temporary stability is achieved by a K-wire and a second positional K-wire is introduced to guide the cannulated screw in right position. **(d–f)** After closed reduction, temporary stability is achieved by a K-wire and a second positional K-wire is introduced to guide the cannulated screw in right position. *(Continued)*

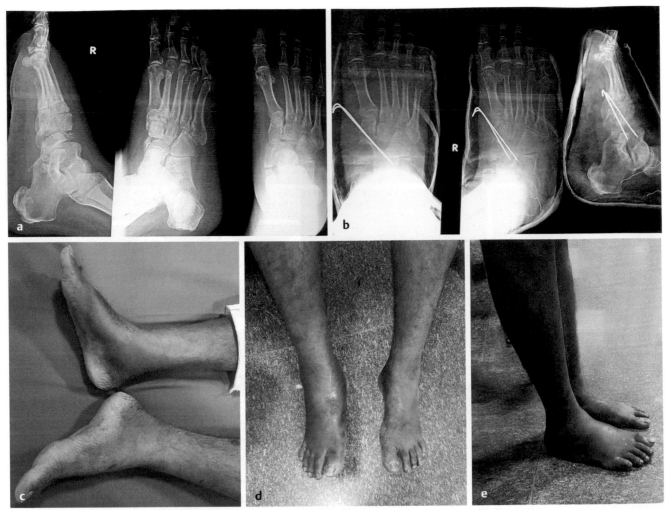

Fig. 14.21 **(a–e)** Naviculocuneiform and talonavicular arthrodesis and fixation with K-wire.

transfixing the joint in reduced position taking into account the medial longitudinal arch. One more horizontal K-wire is added from the base of first metatarsal to second metatarsal shaft in the desired direction as shown in **Fig. 14.22a–e**. One should take into account the transverse arch of the foot while drilling transversely and should feel piercing the first and second cortices of first metatarsal, the third cortex entry on second metatarsal cortex, and the fourth cortex piercing the far cortex of the second metatarsal. This feel is necessary to be absolutely sure about the fixation.

If while inserting the transverse K-wire after exiting the first metatarsal, one is not able to hit the second metatarsal cortex, one can manipulate the second metatarsal by manually raising or lowering the arch to negotiate

and pierce the second metatarsal or by changing the entry point on first metatarsal.

Case Scenario 2

Fracture base of first metatarsal with dorsal subluxation (**Fig. 14.23a–f**). This fracture subluxation is reduced by traction of the big toe and direct pressure over the dorsum of the base of first metatarsal. Two K-wires are passed in similar fashion for fixation of first tarsometatarsal joint (TMTJ) dislocation, one transfixing the medial cuneiform-metatarsal joint and another from the first to second metatarsal base as shown in **Fig. 14.23a–f**. These wires are maintained for a period of 6 weeks and then arch support footwear with partial weight-bearing is started.

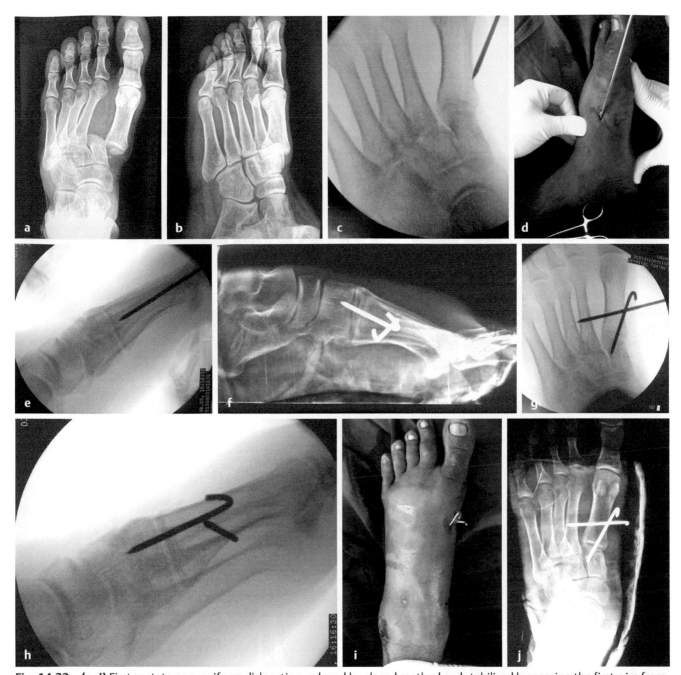

Fig. 14.22 (a–j) First metatarsocuneiform dislocation reduced by closed method and stabilized by passing the first wire from the base of first metatarsal medially angulating up along the arch to transfix the navicular bone in more acute angle (almost parallel to first metatarsal) and the second wire is passed from the base transversely into the second metatarsal (four cortex fixation) as shown.

Lisfranc Fracture Dislocation

Lisfranc Lines (Fig. 14.25a, b)

- In anteroposterior view, medial border of the second metatarsal should be collinear with the medial border of middle cuneiform.
- In oblique view, medial border of fourth metatarsal should be collinear with medial border of cuboid.

Closed manipulation and reduction is done by traction and supination of the forefoot and sometimes with direct pressure over the metatarsal base to relocate the joint. After closed reduction, the position is maintained by two different ways of K-wiring. AP and true lateral views are important to assess the adequacy of reduction.

Method 1: Joint Tansfixation with Oblique K-Wires

Here once the dislocation is reduced, short oblique K-wires are inserted from medial and lateral rays transfixing tarsometatarsal joint to maintain the reduction and alignment. From first metatarsal, medial K-wire is passed about 1 cm away from the tarsometatarsal joint from distal to proximal direction, 70-degree oblique to the first metatarsal in midmedial plane, in order to transfix and secure the tip of the wire into the tarsal bone. Similarly from the fifth metatarsal, lateral K-wire is passed about 1 cm distal to the base of the metatarsal from midlateral plane, distal to proximal direction in 70-degree obliquity to fifth metatarsal, in order to transfix the tarsometatarsal joint as shown in **Fig. 14.26a–g**. An additional transverse K-wire is passed to secure both the columns like a tie beam.

Method 2: Joint Transfixation with Intramedullary K-Wires

The following example (**Fig. 14.27a–e**) shows fracture of the body of medial cuneiform with fracture dislocation of second, third, fourth, and fifth tarsometatarsal joints and lateral displacement.

Lateral view shows dorsal dislocation of the tarsometatarsal joint. From the sole, longitudinal K-wires are passed through the metatarsal head into the shaft and

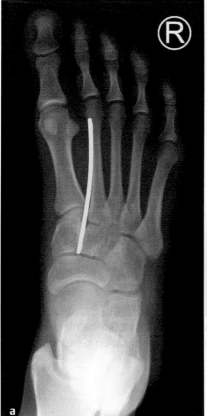

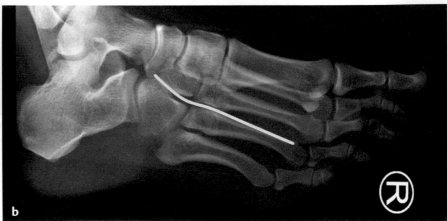

Fig. 14.25 **(a, b)** Lisfranc lines (anteroposterior [AP] and oblique X-ray views). **(a)** In AP view: (1) Lateral border of first metatarsal should be collinear with lateral border of medial cuneiform. (2) Medial border of second metatarsal should be collinear with medial border of middle cuneiform. **(b)** Oblique view: (1) Medial border of fourth metatarsal should be collinear with medial border of cuboid.

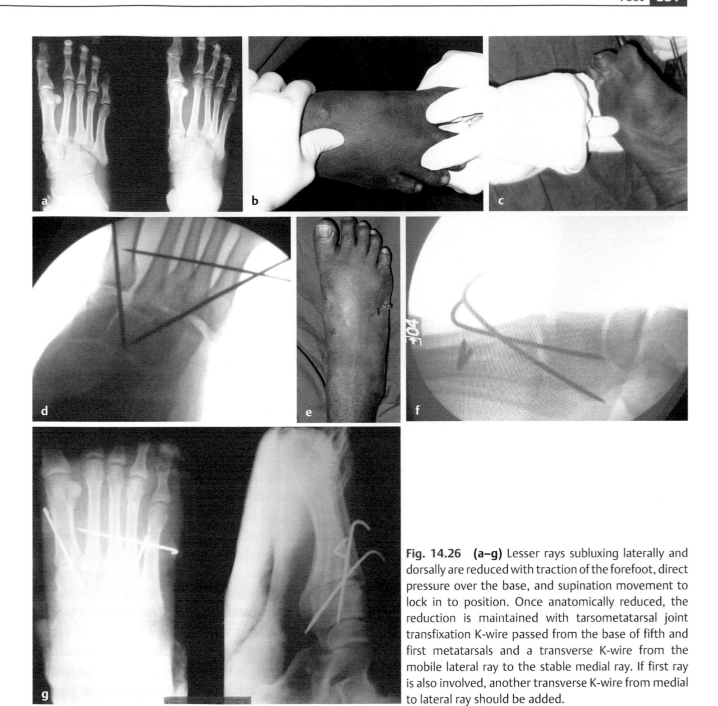

Fig. 14.26 **(a–g)** Lesser rays subluxing laterally and dorsally are reduced with traction of the forefoot, direct pressure over the base, and supination movement to lock in to position. Once anatomically reduced, the reduction is maintained with tarsometatarsal joint transfixation K-wire passed from the base of fifth and first metatarsals and a transverse K-wire from the mobile lateral ray to the stable medial ray. If first ray is also involved, another transverse K-wire from medial to lateral ray should be added.

these K-wires are negotiated through tarsometatarsal joint to transfix through the corresponding tarsals after closed reduction.

Charcot Neuropathic Foot Resulting in Midfoot Break from Lisfranc Fracture Dislocation (Fig. 14.28a–i)

Fracture subluxation of tarsometatarsal joint is one of the common presentations in diabetic neuropathy. In early stages with no displacement, total contact plaster followed by total contact footwear until the stage of remodeling (9–12 months) stops the progression and aids healing. If it progresses like the case shown here, it results in midfoot break causing medial arch support collapse with splaying and lateral subluxation of the forefoot (planovalgus). Patient presents with trophic ulcer over the midfoot medial aspect because of the bony prominence and rocker bottom sole. Debridement of the

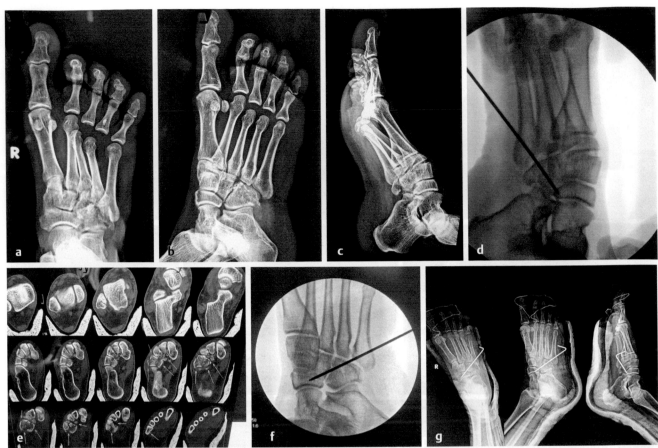

Fig. 14.29 (a–g) Closed reduction and third and fourth metatarsophalangeal dislocation achieved with direct transfixation K-wire due to cuboid fracture.

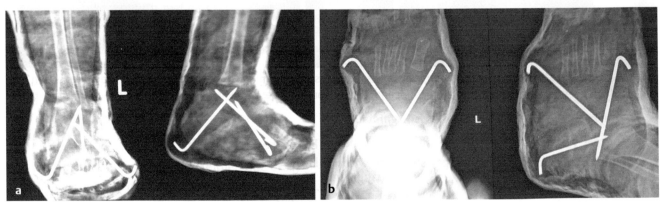

Fig. 14.30 (a, b) In club foot correction by posteromedial release, the talonavicular joint is reduced and transfixed under direct vision with the first K-wire from the navicular bone into the talus, the subtalar joint is everted and pinned from the heel and third wire transfixing the forefoot from lateral ray to midtarsal joint correcting the adduction.

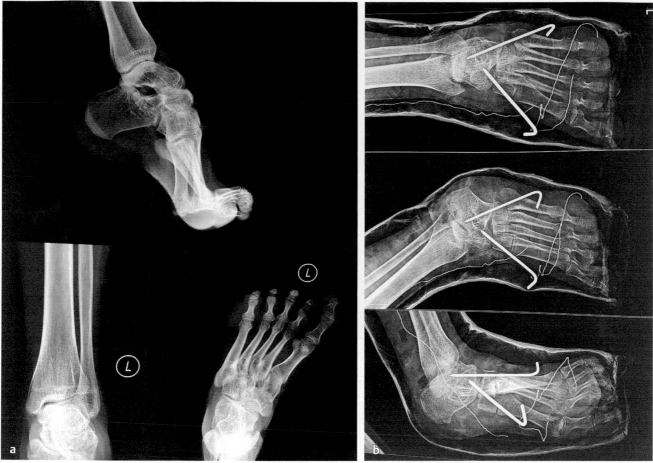

Fig. 14.31 **(a, b)** Dorsolateral closing wedge osteotomy transfixation with K-wiring.

the track. By manual to-and-fro rotation and axial pressure, the K-wire tends to follow the least resistant path (i.e., the medullary canal) to the fracture site. The segmental fracture fragments are manipulated by direct pressure and the wire is passed into the position in fourth and fifth metatarsals transfixing through the cuboid. Here, the third metatarsal is not fixed because of contamination and loss of soft tissue cover (**Fig. 14.33a–c**).

Displaced Second, Third, and Fourth Metatarsal Neck and Head Fracture (Fig. 14.34a, b)

This is treated by retrograde K-wire from the head of metatarsal from plantar aspect. Once the K-wire is centered in the metatarsal head in AP, lateral, and oblique views, it is entered in the distal fragment. K-wire fixing

the head is used like a joystick to reduce the head on to the shaft of the metatarsal and passed intramedullary up to the base of metatarsal securing the reduction.

Displaced First, Second, Third, and Fifth Metetarsal Shaft Fracture (Fig. 14.35a, b and Video 14.1)

These fractures need perfect reduction for effective function of foot as a tripod by maintaining the length and alignment. A retrograde intramedullary K-wire from the plantar aspect of metatarsal head centering on the head, shaft, and base has led to proper alignment and perfect reduction. The K-wires are removed at the end of 5 weeks and assisted weight bearing is started from the end of 6 weeks postoperative.

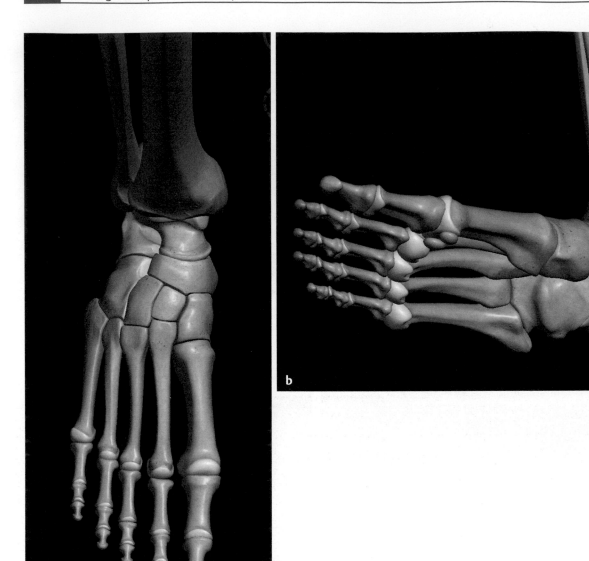

Fig. 14.32   (a, b) Anatomy of the metatarsal articular surface.

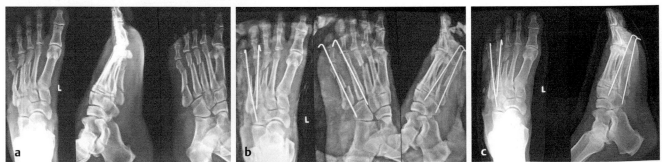

Fig. 14.33   (a, b) K-wire centering the medullary canal in anteroposterior and lateral views is entered through the metatarsal head in the plantar aspect, and once entered, the plier is used to advance the wire forward into the medullary canal and fracture reduced anatomically without any tilt and the wire is transfixed to tarsal bone. **(c)** K-wire centering the medullary canal in anteroposterior and lateral views is entered through the metatarsal head in the plantar aspect, and once entered, the plier is used to advance the wire forward in the medullary canal and fracture reduced anatomically without any tilt and the wire transfixed to tarsal bone.

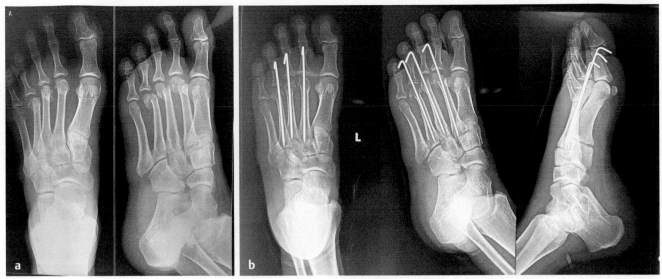

Fig. 14.34 **(a, b)** Second, third, and fourth metatarsal neck fracture treated with intramedullary K-wire.

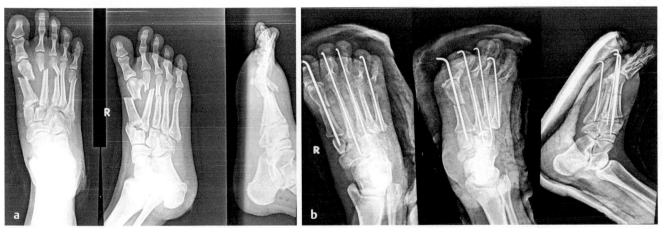

Fig. 14.35 **(a, b)** Retrograde intramedullary K-wire from the plantar aspect of metatarsal head fixing first, second, third, and fifth metatarsal shaft fracture.

Multiple Metatarsal Neck Fracture in a 16-Year-Old Girl (Fig. 14.36a–h)

Undisplaced fracture second and third metatarsal and fourth metatarsal neck fracture with displacement. This is treated with retrograde K-wire from the head of fourth metatarsal plantar aspect, reducing the fracture and negotiating through the medullary canal. It is parked in the tarsal bone for better hold and purchase. A below-knee POP slab is applied for a period of 4 weeks and then

K-wire is removed. Full weight-bearing mobilization is done at the end of 6 weeks.

Fifth Metatarsal Open Fracture with Loss of Bone

The length of the fifth metatarsal is maintained by transfixation transverse K-wire starting from the fifth metatarsal neck to fourth metatarsal shaft as shown in **Fig. 14.37**.

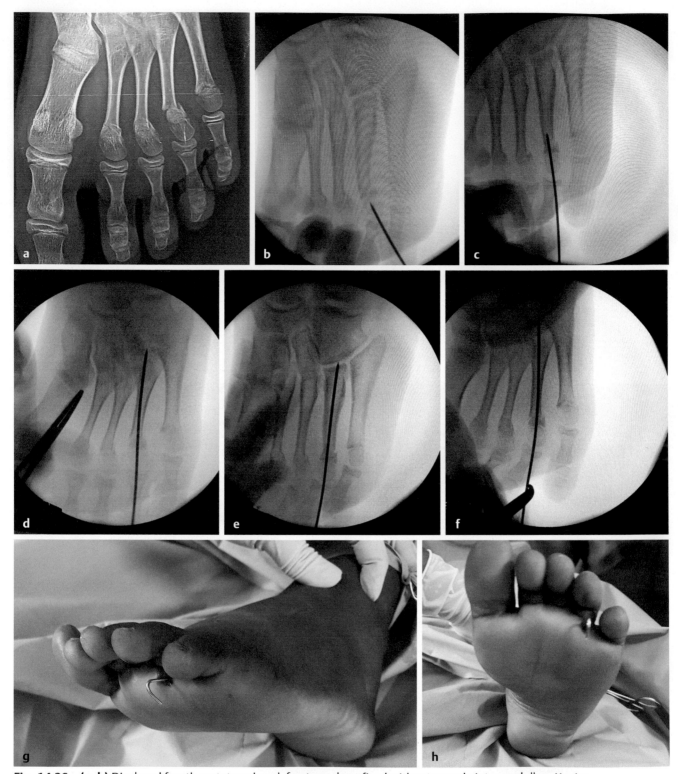

Fig. 14.36 **(a–h)** Displaced fourth metatarsal neck fracture alone fixed with retrograde intramedullary K-wire.

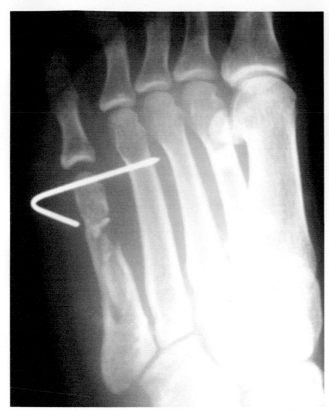

Fig. 14.37 A transverse K-wire is used to span the length out of the fifth metatarsal by transfixing the fifth metatarsal neck to the fourth metatarsal shaft.

Comminuted Fifth Metatarsal Fracture (Fig. 14.38)

Comminution with shortening of fifth metatarsal may affect the tripod load-bearing principle of the foot. The maintenance of length of the lateral column is important for even-load transmission. This is achieved here by reducing the displaced shaft fracture of fifth metatarsal by intramedullary K-wire placement. The wire is passed from the base of the fifth metatarsal in antegrade manner, after previous drilling the lateral cortex with 3.2-mm drill bit for entry. The dorsolateral entry through the opening made with the drill bit is negotiated with 2-mm K-wire whose tip is slightly prebent and the sharp tip is sometimes cut to prevent getting stuck on the inner wall of the medullary canal. By gentle twisting to-and-fro rotary movements, the wire is progressed forward in the medullary canal with a cannulated plier. The prebent tip is twisted accordingly to enter the

medullary canal of distal fragment by closed reduction and manipulation. In this case, there is still some translation and shortening after single-wire placement. Another K-wire of 1.5 mm is inserted to stack the medullary canal and is inserted in the same manner. This technique prevents lateral translation and is able to maintain the length of the metatarsal by parking both the wires at subchondral level keeping the fracture site in distraction. The rotary to-and-fro movement is stopped well before the final position of the wire in the distal fragment. The final parking position of the wire is done by gentle hammering to have an anchorage on the dense subchondral bone and this also prevents loosening or swiveling of the wire.

Hallux Valgus Correction—Chevron Osteotomy (Fig. 14.39)

Many osteotomies of first metatarsal either distal or proximal have been described for hallux valgus correction. The osteotomy can be held in desired position without loss of correction with a simple K-wire fixation and additional plaster boot cast. In the example, a chevron distal metatarsal osteotomy and lateral displacement of the distal head fragment toward the second ray is done to correct the hallux valgus, and bunionectomy is done. A dorsal K-wire is passed transfixing the osteotomy site maintaining good correction for a period of 6 weeks.

Developmental Hallux Valgus (Fig. 14.40)

A 17-year-old girl had progressive big toe deformity from her childhood with hallux valgus and pain in the plantar aspect. X-ray showed hypoplasia of proximal phalanx head radial aspect with fragmentation causing hallux valgus at interphalangeal joint level and a plantar bunion. This is corrected by arthrodesis of interphalangeal joint (IPJ) by denuding the cartilage and levelling the joint to normal alignment and excising the plantar bunion from the base of distal phalanx. Three K-wires are used starting with intramedullary 2-mm K-wire from distal phalanx to proximal phalanx to give normal alignment. Subsequently cross K-wires of 1 mm diameter are used from the sides to transfix the arthrodesis site keeping it in compression mode to maintain static

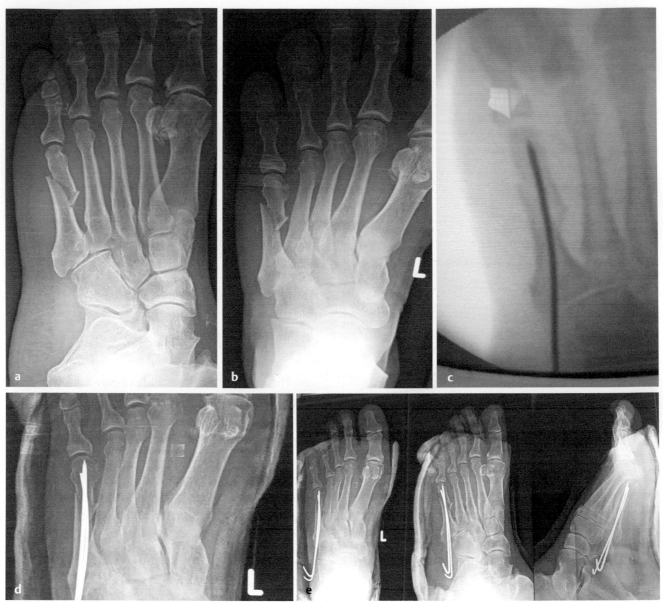

Fig. 14.38 **(a–e)** Fifth metatarsal comminuted fracture with shortening is reduced by stacking two intramedullary K-wires from the base.

compression for fusion. A plaster shoe is used to protect the fusion site for 6 weeks and K-wires are retained for 12 weeks for a solid radiological fusion.

Hallux Flexus—Deformity Correction (Figs. 14.41 and 14.42)

Posttraumatic stiffness with deformity of the great toe causing a nonhealing ulcer on the tip of the toe, due to hallux flexus deformity, is corrected by partial phalangectomy of the base of proximal phalanx (PPX). The deformity is fully corrected. This excision arthroplasty is maintained in anatomical position of 20-degree dorsiflexion from the floor and 7-degree valgus. This is achieved by passing a K-wire in an antegrade manner into the PPX shaft and distal phalanx (DPX), and then in retrograde insertion into the metatarsal head.

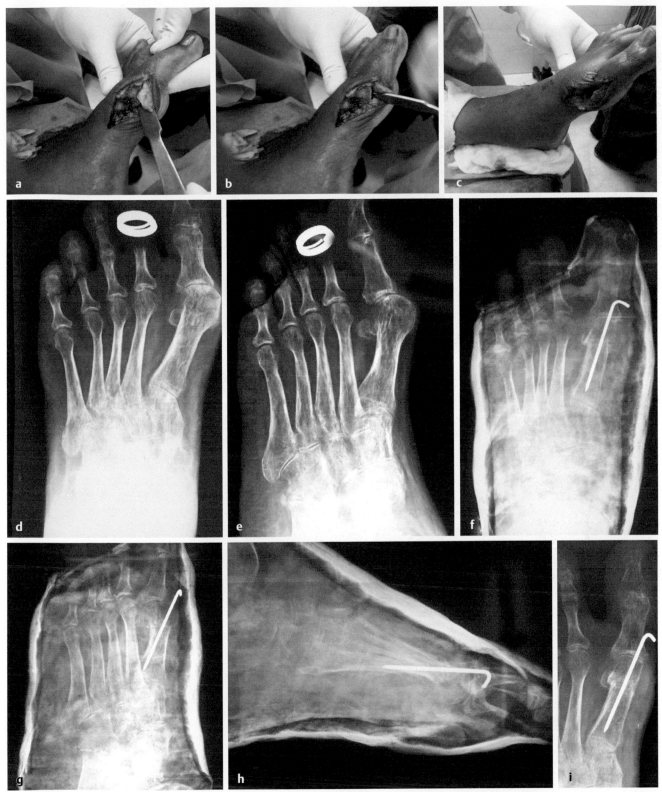

Fig. 14.39 **(a–i)** First metatarsal head displacement chevron osteotomy is transfixed with single K-wire for prevention of loss of position by direct anchoring through the metatarsal head dorsomedially.

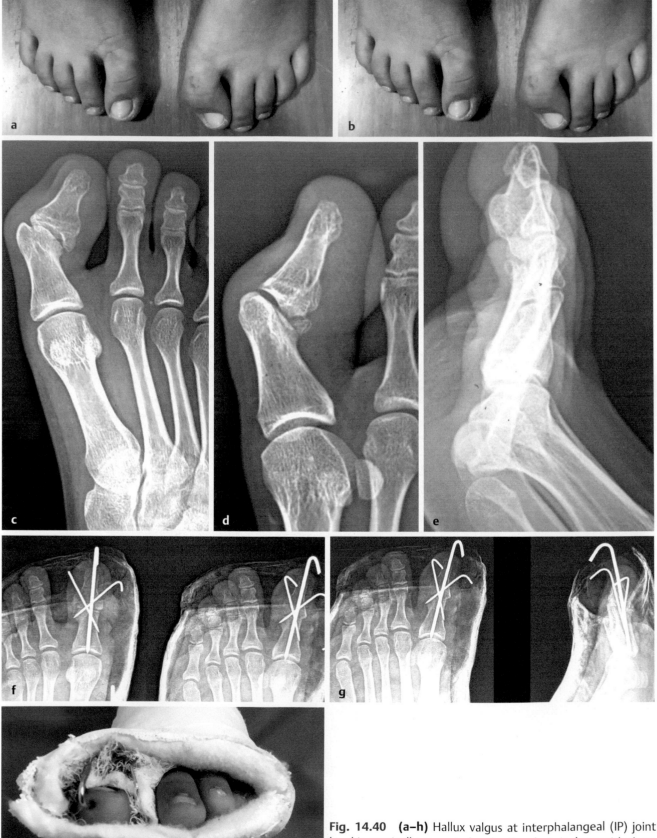

Fig. 14.40 (a–h) Hallux valgus at interphalangeal (IP) joint level is surgically corrected and arthrodesis is done with three K-wire technique.

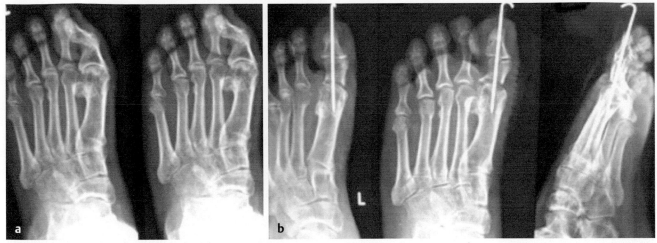

Fig. 14.41 **(a, b)** After hallux flexus correction, the reduction is maintained by passing an ante/retrograde K-wire through the proximal phalanx base and wire passed back through the metatarsal head in 20-degree dorsiflexion and 7-degree valgus maintaining it for 6 weeks.

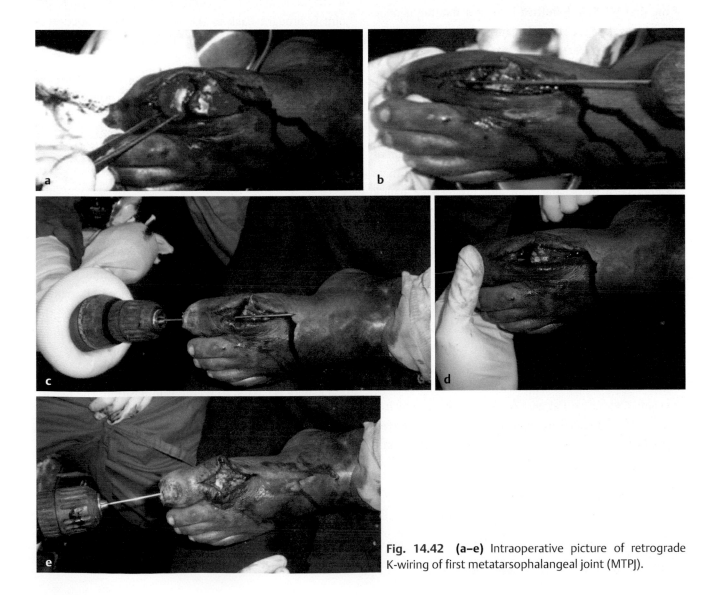

Fig. 14.42 **(a–e)** Intraoperative picture of retrograde K-wiring of first metatarsophalangeal joint (MTPJ).

Hallux Rigidus—First Metatarsophalangeal Arthrodesis (Fig. 14.43a–e)

Arthritic first MTPJ is fused to alleviate pain and give strength on push-off at stance phase. The ideal position of fusion is 10-degree dorsiflexion to the floor and 10-degree valgus. This procedure is done by dorsal approach. After the cartilage is denuded, the MTPJ is fixed temporarily by a K-wire in the desired angle of fusion of 10-degree valgus and 10-degree of dorsiflexion of the PPX in respect to the floor. A K-wire is passed from distal to proximal from the PPX base obliquely pointing to the plantar medial surface transfixing first MTP eccentrically in good approximation and alignment. This K-wire would not be hindering the way of definitive fixation by a lag screw which will pass in the center of the first MTPJ. A definitive lag screw fixation is done from the neck of metatarsal at medial-plantar aspect to PPX shaft as the direction is desirable for fixation in good alignment and for good compression. K-wire is removed before final tightening of the lag screw.

Bifid Big Toe with Hallux Varus (Fig. 14.44a–j)

It is a congenital condition with complete duplication of PPX and DPX from first MTPJ level. A 28-year-old male presents with increasing pain and progressive hallux varus deformity for past few months. Patient has excision of the medial most rudimentary big toe and hallux varus is addressed by correcting the metatarsal articular surface slope with first metatarsal dome osteotomy and achieving the normal valgus of 7 degrees. A horizontal K-wire parallel to the joint surface of first metatarsal is inserted from medial side and it is used to lever the joint perpendicular to the shaft. Once correction is achieved an oblique K-wire from metatarsal head is inserted to transfix the osteotomy site and anchored on the shaft. The horizontal wire used in the head, which is used to lever the head fragment, is subsequently driven in, to anchor on the second metatarsal for additional stability.

Trophic Ulcer Big Toe Plantar Side (Fig. 14.45a–m)

Infected trophic ulcer is excised and it communicates to IPJ with osteomyelitic changes. Excision of the infected

PPX head is performed with thorough debridement. To achieve stability antegrade K-wire is passed from the base of DPX through the wound and retrograde insertion back into the remaining PPX and transfixation on metatarsal head is done. The wire is maintained for 6 weeks for good soft tissue healing and stability.

Big Toe Injury

Old Unreduced First Metatarsophalangeal Joint Dislocation (Fig. 14.46a–d)

An initially failed closed manipulation is left untreated for 4 weeks duration, resulting in open reduction. In this case, the metatarsal head is buttonholed through the plantar plate in between the sesamoids. After one of the sesamoids is excised by dorsal approach, the joint is brought back to the position. The reduction is maintained by percutaneous K-wire passed from the PPX base from medial side directed toward the first metatarsal head in order to transfix the joint. This is maintained for a period of 6 weeks with additional POP cast support.

Partial Intra-Articular Fracture Head of Proximal Phalanx Big Toe

Avulsion Fracture Lateral Condyle Head of Proximal Phalanx Big Toe (Fig. 14.47a–d)

Avulsion fracture of the lateral condyle head of PPX with rotation and displacement is due to varus injury to the big toe. This displaced fragment is reduced by maneuvering with a K-wire as shown in **Fig. 14.47a–d**, and the articular surface is matched. Sometimes an open reduction may be necessary if the fragment does not fall in place. Once the fragment is in congruity, a fragment fixation K-wire is passed to secure it in position. The K-wire is retained for a period of 6 weeks.

Avulsion Fracture Medial Condyle Head of Proximal Phalanx Big Toe (Fig. 14.48 a–c)

Medial condyle fracture of the PPX head with displacement and rotation is corrected and transfixed with oblique K-wire. Though it is suboptimal in reduction, the joint alignment and stability is good and has good functional result in follow-up. Sometimes if the

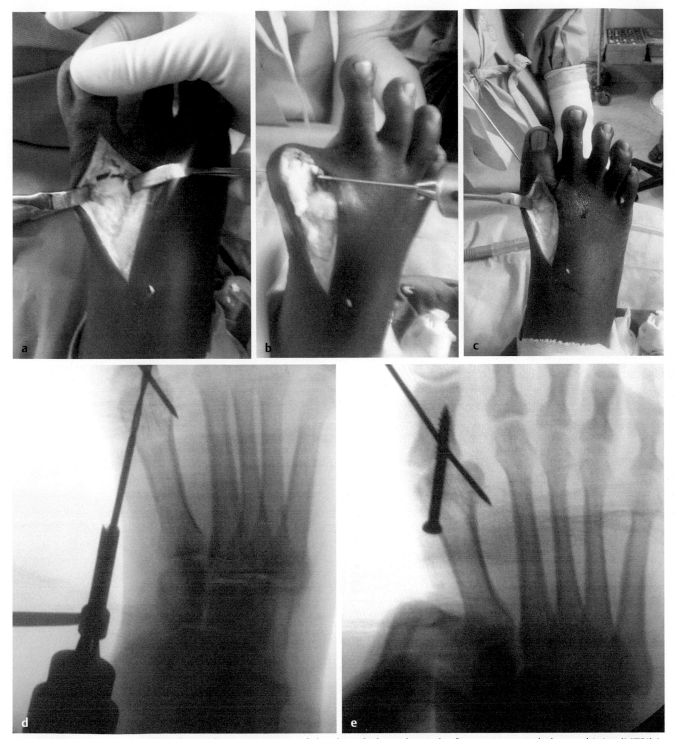

Fig. 14.43 **(a–e)** Open arthrodesis after preparation of the denuded cartilage; the first metatarsophalangeal joint (MTPJ) is aligned and fixed with a temporary K-wire such that it does not come in the way of definitive fixation with a lag screw as shown.

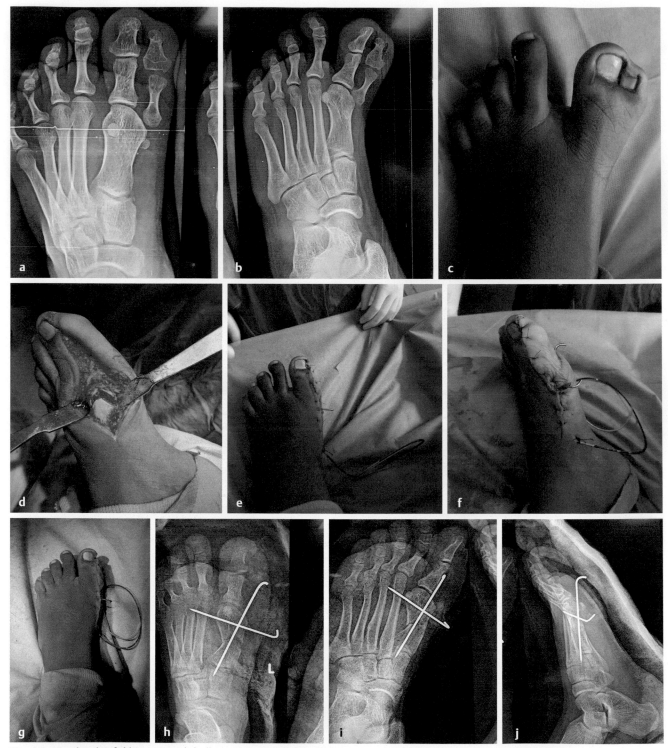

Fig. 14.44 **(a–j)** Bifid big toe with hallux varus correction with intermetatarsal dome osteotomy and K-wire stabilization.

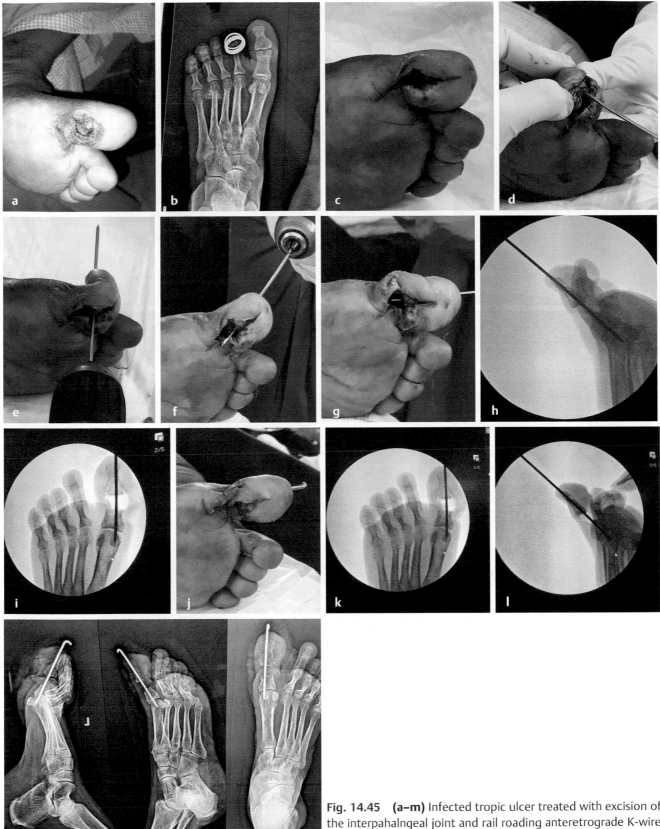

Fig. 14.45 **(a–m)** Infected tropic ulcer treated with excision of the interpahalngeal joint and rail roading anteretrograde K-wire fixation to stabilize resection arthroplasty.

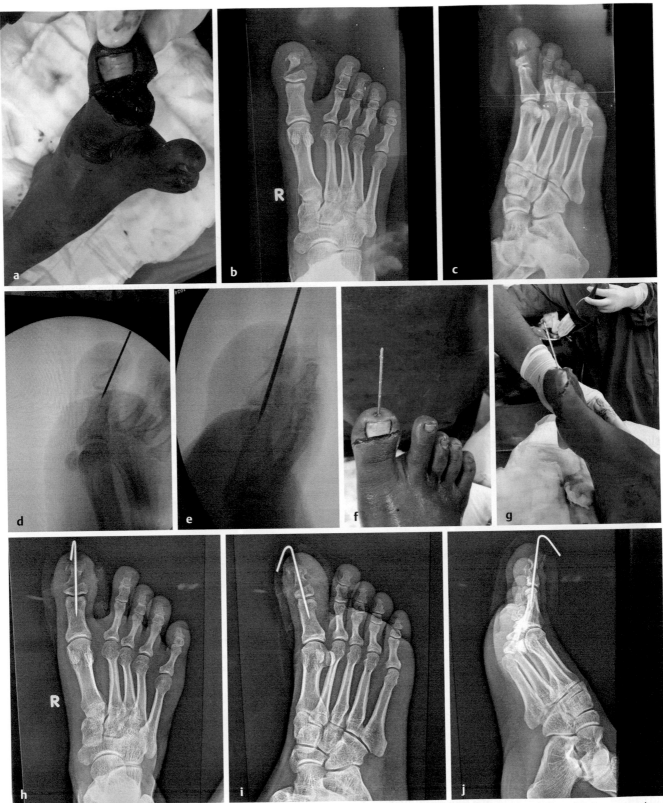

Fig. 14.55 (a–j) Open distal phalanx fracture terated with retrograde intramedullary K-wiring and parking on proximal phalanx head for stability.

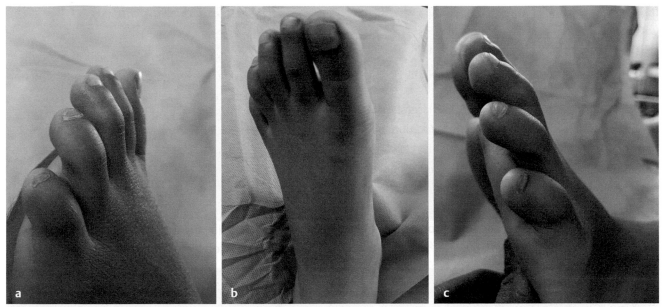

Fig. 14.56 (a–c) Attitude of the toes: slight dorsiflexion at the metatarsophalangeal joint (MTPJ), slight flexion at the proximal interphalangeal joint (PIPJ) and straight neutral position of the distal interphalangeal joint (DIPJ).

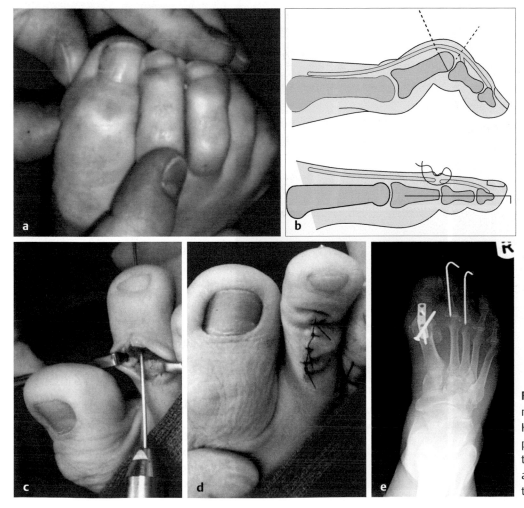

Fig. 14.57 (a–e) Ante/retrograde passing of K-wire through the middler phalanx base and back into the proximal phalanx (PPX) after excision arthroplasty to correct the deformity.

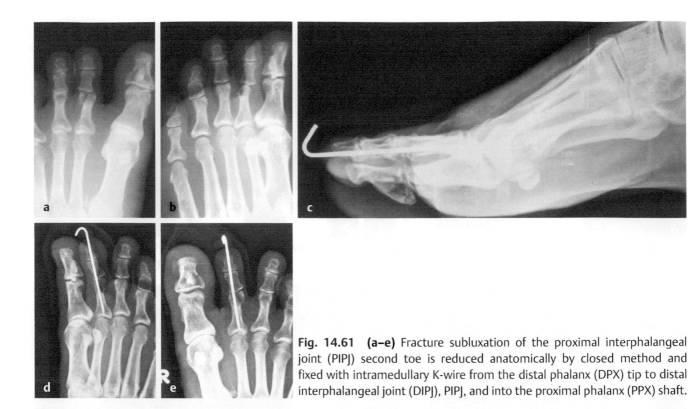

Fig. 14.61 (a–e) Fracture subluxation of the proximal interphalangeal joint (PIPJ) second toe is reduced anatomically by closed method and fixed with intramedullary K-wire from the distal phalanx (DPX) tip to distal interphalangeal joint (DIPJ), PIPJ, and into the proximal phalanx (PPX) shaft.

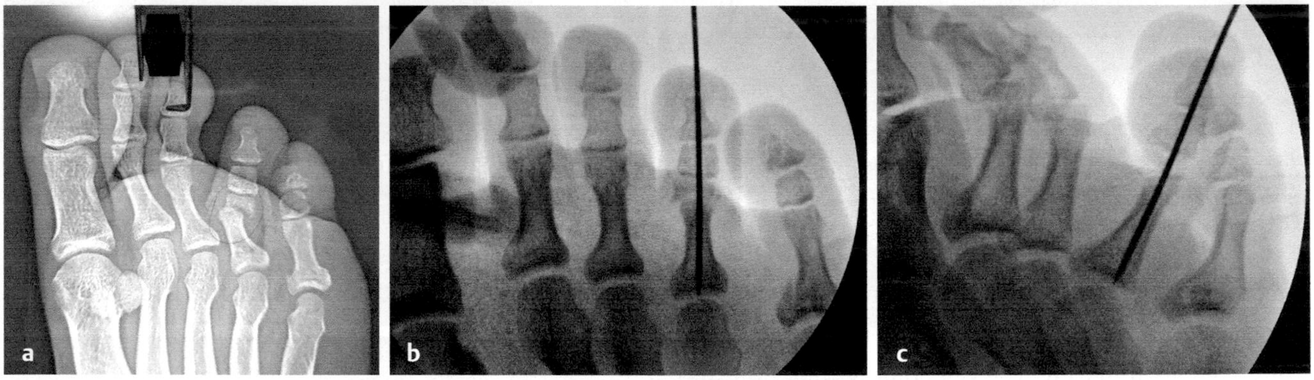

Fig. 14.62 (a–c) The fourth toe proximal phalanx (PPX) is fixed with intramedullary K-wire from the head of PPX retrograde and parking at the base of PPX. The adjacent fifth toe is treated with buddy strapping.

Little Toe Injury

Physeal Separation of Proximal Phalanx Little Toe with Displacement (Salter-Harris Type II) (Fig. 14.64a, b)

A percutaneous K-wire fixation is done after reduction of the fracture with two K-wires transfixing the physis, without crossing the MTPJ. This is passed after closed reduction of fracture by traction and adduction of the fifth toe. K-wire is passed from lateral aspect close to physis, distal to proximal, transfixing the physeal fracture. Sometimes the first wire after piercing the PPX shaft can be used as a joystick to manipulate, reduce, and then to transfix across the epiphysis. The second wire is used to give rotational stability and also to ensure that if the first wire does not give good hold and in right

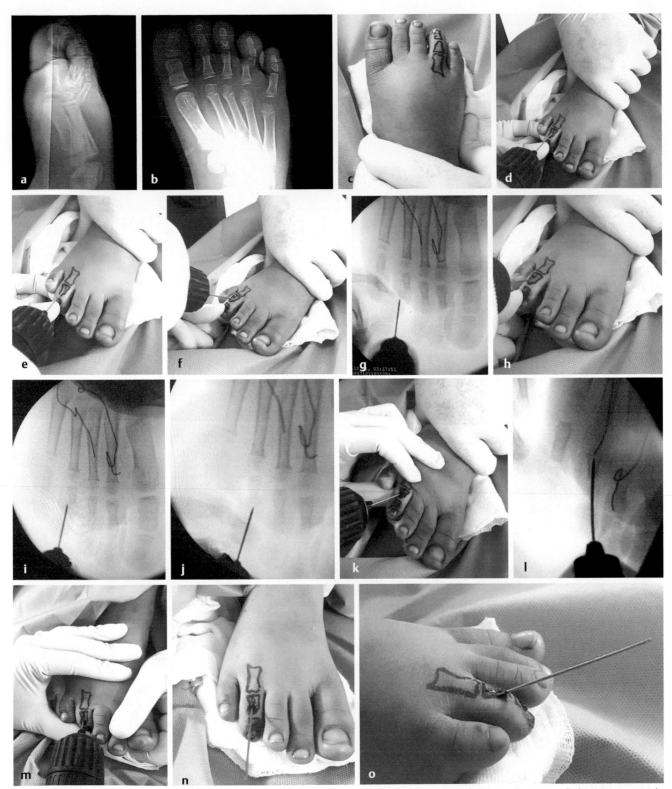

Fig. 14.63 (a–o) The surface marking indicates the position of the phalanges and the technique of direct retrograde intramedullary K-wire fixation from the PPX neck fracture through head of PPX.

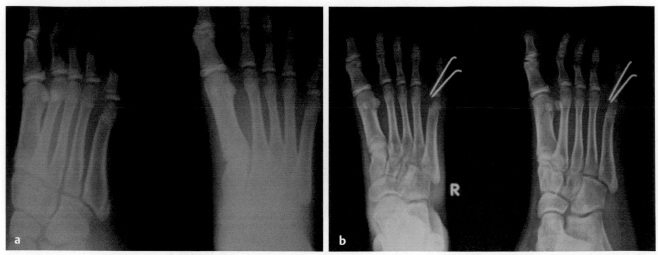

Fig. 14.64 **(a, b)** Fifth toe physeal fracture with displacement of the proximal phalanx (PPX) is reduced and transfixed with two K-wires from the shaft to epiphysis.

position, this wire would do the trick. In this case, one wire is eccentric in the fixation of epiphysis and hence an additional K-wire is inserted to ensure that there is no loss of fixation.

Fracture of Proximal Phalanx Base of Fifth Toe (Fig. 14.65a–g)

Any fracture of PPX in the toe tends to hyperextend to cause an angular deformity along with rotation. One needs to correct the dorsal tilt, angulation, and rotation of the distal fragment. Normally the MTPJ is dorsiflexed (30–40 degrees), and to reduce this fracture, one should give longitudinal traction with flexion at the IPJ and MTPJ to correct excessive dorsiflexion. After position is checked with C-arm scan, K-wire is passed dorsally from the PPX head in a flexed PIPJ position. Straight intramedullary wire centering in AP/lateral view transfixing the fracture from distal to proximal fragment is passed. In extreme comminution of PPX base, it is advisable to transfix into the metatarsal head maintaining the length and the normal dorsiflexed position of the toe (**Fig. 14.65a–g**).

Open Fifth Toe Proximal Phalanx Fracture (Fig. 14.66a–g)

This is a quite common fracture of little toe with open web space laceration between the fourth and fifth toe. Here it is foot pedal injury from a motor bike collision.

After thorough debridement of the fifth toe, PPX is reduced and fixed with retrograde K-wire from the PIPJ through the head of PPX intramedullary through the fracture and parked on the head of fifth metatarsal bone in the dorsiflexed position. This wire is left in for a period of 4 weeks with heel weight-bearing mobilization. The wire is subsequently removed and rehabilitation exercises are done.

Unstable PIPJ Dislocation Fifth Toe (Fig. 14.67a–d)

A closed domestic injury to the fifth toe by striking accidentally against an object resulted in subluxation of PIPJ. The closed reduction under digit block anesthesia is done but it remains unstable. Hence an oblique K-wire transfixing the PIPJ from middle phalanx base to PPX is passed maintaining the congruity.

Open Dislocation of Proximal Interphalangeal Joint of Little Toe (Fig. 14.68a–c)

In side swipe injury from a motorbike accident, the little toe fracture or open dislocation is common with web space laceration. In this case, the open dislocation was debrided and then reduced. The dislocation was unstable and strapping to the neighboring fourth toe couldnot be done because of web space wound which required regular dressing. The PIPJ was hence transfixed in anatomical congruency by a transfixing K-wire from the side in an oblique fashion as shown in **Fig. 14.68a–c**.

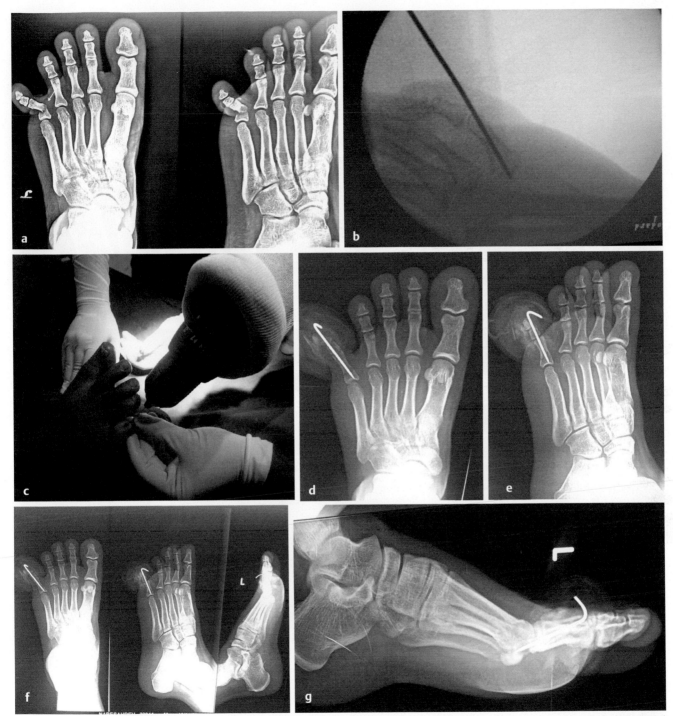

Fig. 14.65 (a–g) Fifth toe displaced fracture is reduced by passing an intramedullary wire from the proximal phalanx (PPX) head to the base.

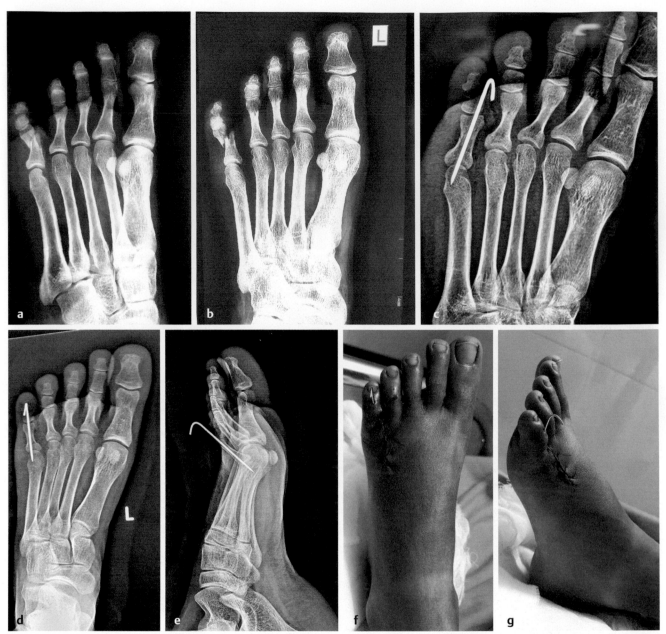

Fig. 14.66 **(a–g)** Open fracture PPX fifth toe debrided and PPX intramedullary K-wire fixation done by retrograde method starting from head of PPX and anchoring on the fifth metatarsal head.

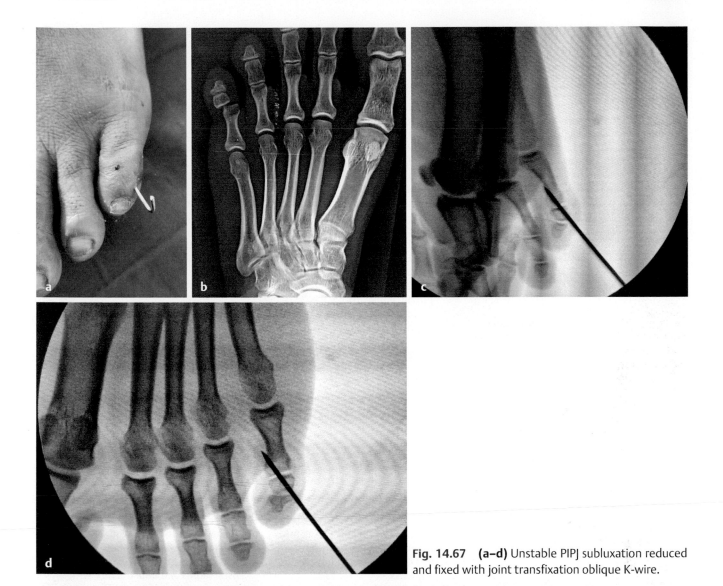

Fig. 14.67 **(a–d)** Unstable PIPJ subluxation reduced and fixed with joint transfixation oblique K-wire.

Fig. 14.68 **(a–c)** After debridement, the proximal interphalangeal joint (PIPJ) was reduced and transfixed with an oblique K-wire from lateral to medial direction from middle phalanx to proximal phalanx (PPX).

Index